PRAISE FOR *THAT TIME I GOT CANCER*

"It is hard to convey how intimate this memoir is, how revealing, and how moving. With unflinching candor and rare introspection, Zervanos takes us on a tour of life's scariest moments, and also of its most redemptive—and we are all improved by this journey he so generously shares. This is a brilliant, important book."

—Robin Black, Author of *Life Drawing*

"Through his extraordinarily written and heartfelt expression, Jim Zervanos speaks for people who have been through this kind of trauma and gives them an opportunity for catharsis and psychic relief. This book will be enjoyed—yes, *enjoyed*—and will be most useful for those who want and need to share in the expression of what they've been through. We can all celebrate and share in the joy of life. Truly, this book will help patients, and every medical student in the country should read it."

—Stephen J. Schuster, MD, Director of the Lymphoma Program at the Hospital of the University of Pennsylvania

"Jim Zervanos has crafted a narrative that feels like something out of Dante, only the paths he circles lead us to an internal inferno: a fire inside his own body. With candor and precision, so much humor and grace, Zervanos leads us through a health emergency he's lucky to have survived—and we're luckier still, having this brilliant account in our hands. This is a memoir you'll want to hand to everyone you know."

—Daniel Torday, Author of Boomer 1

"Zervanos has managed to capture the very difficult decisions doctors face every day, as well as the importance of patient involvement in decision-making. I have used his case in teaching generations of residents the value of restraint in treatment, of recognizing the crucial difference between what we *can* do and what we *should* do. Moreover, Zervanos conveys how illness affects both the patient and the entire family. As physicians, we often fail to appreciate this impact, as does anyone who has not been through the illness of a family member. As I read his story, I felt his pain as well as his family's pain, and I felt the relief and rejuvenation of his recovery and growth."

—Scott O. Trerotola, MD, Associate Chair and Chief, Interventional Radiology, Department of Radiology, Perelman School of Medicine at the University of Pennsylvania

That Time I Got Cancer: A Love Story

by Jim Zervanos

ISBN 978-1-64663-817-8

Published by

◄ köehlerbooks™

3705 Shore Drive
Virginia Beach, VA 23455
800-435-4811
www.koehlerbooks.com

THAT TIME I GOT CANCER

— A LOVE STORY —

JIM ZERVANOS

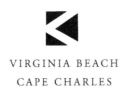

VIRGINIA BEACH
CAPE CHARLES

*To my family and friends
and to Dr. Alberto Pochettino, Dr. Stephen Schuster,
and Dr. Scott Trerotola and to all the doctors, nurses, and supporting staff
at the Hospital of the University of Pennsylvania*

We come from a dark abyss, we end in a dark abyss,
and we call the luminous interval life.

—Nikos Kazantzakis

TABLE OF CONTENTS

Seeing Stars 1

Part I 5

    1. Young and Hip 7

    2. Home Again 10

    3. Bethany Beach 18

    4. The Bear 25

    5. Labor Day Weekend 31

    6. The Helmet 40

    7. Doomsday 44

    8. Hail Mary 50

    9. Big Brother 55

    10. Communion 60

    11. Awake 68

    12. The Diagnosis 75

Part II 83

    13. Tree of Life 85

    14. Grafts and Stents and Chemotherapy 90

    15. The Rise of Cancer Boy 108

    16. Happy Birthday 114

    17. Outta Here 120

    18. Testosterone 124

    19. Merry Christmas and Happy New Year 130

    20. Prednisone 136

21. Things We're Looking Forward To 139

22. Quarantine 142

Part III 153

23. Heaven on Earth 155

24. Once More Unto the Breach, Dear Friends 160

25. Psycho-Social Acceleration 173

26. Thank You for Saving My Life, by the Way 181

27. He's All I've Got, She Said 187

28. Angioplasty 193

29. Night Sweats 199

30. Anniversary 205

Begin Again 208

Acknowledgments 213

SEEING STARS

In the early afternoon of an otherwise idyllic October Saturday, I braced myself against the kitchen table, suddenly dizzy, vision clouded, head swelling with surging blood as if I were being strangled from the inside. It had been five years since my illness, but these familiar symptoms could still be brought on by physical stress—and, as it turned out, extreme emotional distress. But never before so intensely as this. On the laptop left open by my wife was an unfinished letter from her to me. *I love you, but...*

The blackout never quite came. I read what remained on the page, composed sometime between last night and an hour ago, before she took our six-year-old to his soccer game, where they were right now. *I can't live like this. We just don't connect anymore...* These words I was not meant to discover—or maybe I was. I closed the laptop, throat clenched, vision clarified, and walked outside into the front yard, drenched in sunlight.

A neighbor stopped on the sidewalk, dog in tow, and called to me on the porch. "Are you okay?" I hadn't realized I was crying so loudly. I waved, and he continued hesitantly on.

I phoned my brother, recently divorced, and told him of what I had just read. "How can she give all this up?"

John kept his cool, told me how things tended to go from here. "No matter what happens," he said, "you've got your family. Your kids. Me and Sue, Mom and Dad. Your amazing friends. You've got all of us behind you."

"I'm not as strong as you," I said.

"Like hell you aren't," he said. "You've been through worse."

I hesitated. "This is *worse* than cancer—"

"Stop—"

I stopped. Still, it seemed true. Somehow losing my life had not felt as bad as losing everything I loved, which was what this felt like right now.

"Don't do anything rash," he said. "You tell her you need space from each other, to think about what's next. You ask her to go home to her parents for the night and come back tomorrow. You're going to get through this."

I took in his instructions faithfully.

From the front yard I stared at our house. I pictured Victor, our two-year-old, the diligent napper, tucked soundly under blankets in his bedroom. I imagined, in a nearby park, Nikitas, our six-year-old, in his little shin guards and soccer shirt with vertical blue stripes, tearing down the field toward the goal. I saw Vana on the sidelines, gorgeous and sad, steely-eyed behind dark sunglasses.

I called my sister, Sue, in Lancaster. "Are you busy?" I asked.

"I'm downtown at the market. What's the matter?"

The tears started again. "I need your help."

"I'm coming," and she was on her way.

Pacing in the grass, I recalled last night, at dusk, when Vana returned from a business trip in New York, our walk around the block, her new posture, the space between us, her hands in her coat pockets. She paused to be sure I was looking at her face when she said she could have flown—gone to the airport and just flown, anywhere, to Boston or California, just away. Vana, who hated flying more than anything. She was done with the old fears and inhibitions.

She'd felt alive in New York. She'd felt like herself, in a way she hadn't felt in a long time, if ever, at least with me. "I've changed," she said.

Now I was gazing up at the blue sky, feeling blindsided. I recalled the love letters doodled with flowers left on my desk. But that was long ago, in a different time and place. How could I have let things come to this? And how could I recover what had been lost?

As she pulled into the driveway, I managed to keep it cool in front of Nikitas. "Go inside, buddy," I said, and he did. She listened to my proposal. "Go to your parents. I'll stay here." She said I wasn't in a state to be alone with the kids. I said my sister was on her way. At last she agreed, packed a bag, and told Nikitas, who was quietly watching cartoons, that she was going home to visit Nana and Pop-Pop and she'd be back in the morning.

That night sitting on the porch I felt strangely calm, staring out at the yard where hours earlier I'd been pacing desperately.

Vana called and said she was in the car, and she was on her way home. "Please don't," I said. "Go back to your mom's. Get some sleep. Wake up tomorrow. Then come back." Back to our house. Back to our kids. Back to *us.* She took a deep breath and turned around again.

I looked out at the bright stars in the dark sky. The porch warmly lit around me. The window glowing behind me. My sister lying on the couch watching TV inside. The kids upstairs sleeping. I breathed in the cold night air.

I was now in my mid-forties, and five years had passed since I'd been sick. I'd believed that life had returned to normal, or even gotten better. Or at least that *my* life had. Only now was I beginning to understand what I—or *we*—had actually been through. *Everything* had changed—because everything is always changing.

I exhaled a long breath. Nothing of the future was certain. This is what I'd learned. Anything can happen anytime.

And then I remembered the words my doctor had spoken when all seemed lost—what I should have known all along. *"There is always hope."* I wanted to believe it still.

PART I

Write as if you were dying. At the same time, assume you write for an audience consisting solely of terminal patients. That is, after all, the case.

—Annie Dillard

There's a darkness on the edge of town.

—Bruce Springsteen

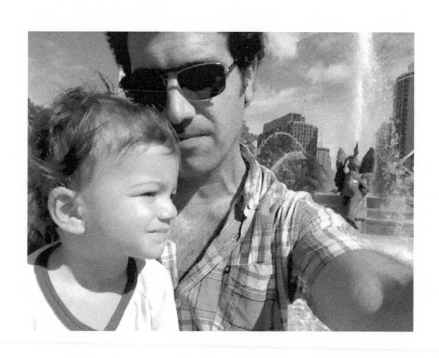

1

YOUNG AND HIP

S itting on the ledge of our favorite fountain, where frogs and swans spouted towers of water, Nikitas and I mugged for selfies after a long afternoon walk.

In an hour, everything would change. Days from now these pictures would seem to come from a life that was no longer mine—or ours.

Nikitas was in profile in the foreground, staring curiously at the world I tried to imagine through his one-year-old eyes. My eyes were behind black sunglasses. My collar was open. The veins on the left side of my neck, highlighted by bold strokes of shade, exuded vitality—or so it seemed.

In that moment, life was perfect. Just an ordinary Tuesday. It really had been the most beautiful day of the summer. Though it was already five o'clock and I would soon be going to the Phillies game with my father-in-law, I couldn't resist the scenic route home. We circled the Rodin Museum, skirted the Barnes Museum construction site, passed the Whole Foods, and paused at the intersection across from Starbucks, where I planned to grab a cup of coffee so that I'd be wide awake for the late innings.

Under the canopy of trees at the corner, two women—one

holding a camera, the other a clipboard—emerged from behind the Whole Foods sign set in the ground near some shrubbery. The two women winked to each other in confirmation. The woman with the camera asked me if I'd be willing to speak with them, answer a few questions, for no more than two minutes. They'd be quick, she said, seeing that I had my little boy with me. They were from Sears, she said, and they were looking for people to be in a national commercial.

She handed me a photocopy with the company logo, below which the marketing scheme was spelled out: *Sears is currently looking for hip, active, and fun men and women of all ethnicities between the ages of 25-35 to audition for a very unique ad campaign!*

"I'm forty-one with a kid," I said. "Neither young nor hip."

She said she would ask me simple questions, just to see how I looked and sounded, while she filmed me. I was delaying, contemplating my hypocrisy and the dishwasher Vana and I swore would be the last thing we would ever buy from Sears, after an excruciating experience trying to return a lemon with a broken latch that sat in our kitchen for months. I signed the contract, agreeing to be filmed, untroubled by my easy willingness to sell my soul for my fifteen minutes—or thirty seconds—to be featured in a TV commercial hawking wares for a company toward which I held a personal grudge.

She asked me to remove my sunglasses. When I did, she gave a pleased glance to her quiet colleague and said, "I think we found our guy." She peppered me with questions.

"Where do you live?"

"What do you do?"

"What are your hobbies?"

"Are you married?"

"How old is your son?"

"Is he always so well behaved?"

As I answered, I was certain my lack of enthusiasm was disappointing these women and dooming my chances. The interviewer told me this was just the kind of cool they were looking for. I thought, *I can't keep this act up for much longer.*

She told me that the commercial would be shot in two weeks. The "actors" would be selected in the next few days. If chosen, I would be paid over five hundred dollars for the day's work. If I were featured prominently and the commercial ran nationally, I could make as much as fifteen thousand dollars. *Not bad,* I thought. This could be fun after all. She told me to expect a call. I shook their hands and went across the street for my coffee. Through the window at Starbucks, I watched the two women in the shadows behind the Whole Foods sign. They appeared to be packing up. I was feeling encouraged, as young hip people passed them by without being snagged.

Walking home, I smiled, understanding that I'd been afforded my fair share of bizarrely wonderful experiences in life. And yet, at that moment, I was most grateful for the daily joys I experienced as a teacher with summers off, for the sunshine through the trees, the pleasant sights and sounds of the city I loved. I laughed, realizing I was at a point in my life, *at last,* where I could take or leave a Sears commercial, the prospects for which felt more like a burden than a lucky break—notwithstanding the checks I wouldn't mind receiving. The new school year would be starting in two weeks, and I'd finally gotten some momentum with the novel I was writing.

The little rendezvous with the talent scouts would suffice for an amusing story, which I was eager to tell Vana and her father, who was on his way to Philadelphia for the game tonight. Doc Halladay would be on the mound against Arizona. The Phils were on track to win a record number of games this season. The forecast promised a perfect summer night.

2

HOME AGAIN

had just taken a shower and was getting dressed to go to the Phillies game when in the mirror I saw my face darkening to purple. I called out to Vana, who rushed upstairs. "Oh my God," she said.

"What's happening to me?"

She watched in speechless terror. In seconds I understood that if this mysterious flooding continued, I would soon witness my own grotesque demise. Downstairs Nikitas was waiting with Vana's father, who had just arrived to drive us to the ballpark.

I decided it was too late to call 911, so I called my dad, a doctor, who, upon hearing my quick description of my symptoms, advised me to take deep breaths, and so I did. I breathed. In. And out. My face swelled with surging blood. As Vana watched, I thought, *I love you*. And, *I might be dying*. My eyes moved back and forth between Vana and the mirror. We waited. The brief time that followed stretched into a kind of eternity. Again and again, I breathed in, and out.

Minutes passed. The flooding subsided. I was breathing easily. *I'm better now*, I told myself. My dad said, "Go to the emergency room. *Now!*"

The fear returned, and, with it, the awe. Of what I had just experienced. Of the unimaginable that was still to come. I looked at

Vana and this space that was home. I took a deep breath and felt alive.

. . .

I was in the emergency room at the University of Pennsylvania, and in a matter of minutes, I was called back for tests. This was the first sign that the symptoms I'd reported to the welcoming nurse were cause for urgent concern. I was given an EKG, and before long I was seated in my own room. Naively, I thought I might still make it to the Phillies game with my father-in-law, who was in the waiting room. By seven o'clock, the attending doctor told me to send my father-in-law on his way; I was going to be here for a while.

I watched the Phils on TV. At 9:30 X-rays were taken. I was given an ultrasound. Later, a hysterical woman was brought in on a wheelchair, rushed down the hallway and into a nearby room, screaming, "I'm dying! Oh, God!" I understood that the ER docs had other priorities. I watched Halladay lose his lead in the ninth.

At 12:30 a CAT-scan was done on my neck and chest. Sometime after that I found Dr. Utley behind the main desk and asked if she was surprised that the test results were not back yet. She gave me a sympathetic look and said she'd come see me in a minute. Back in my room, she held the black-and-white CAT-scan image.

"See this?" She pointed.

Two fuzzy gray bands appeared strangely narrowed. These were the crucial veins to the heart, she explained. She tilted her head sadly. "This could be fatal. We just don't know what this is."

I took in the words.

She leaned forward, as if to hug me. I wanted her to.

. . .

I sat alone in a frozen fog. Tuesday had become Wednesday. Hours had passed since I'd spoken to anyone in my family. I couldn't bring myself to pick up the phone, much less to provide an update. At 2:30 a.m. I was wheeled to the basement for an MRI. Inside the tube I kept my cool by thinking of Nikitas, the two of us just hours ago at our favorite fountain, drenched in sunshine.

Back in my room, I gathered my wits and called Vana, whose sleepless voice soothed me. Despite her compounding fears, she managed to hide behind her sympathetic expressions. *I'm sorry I'm not there with you. You must be so scared.* I spared her the words that Dr. Utley had said to me: *This could be fatal.* I imagined Vana alone in our oversized bed, trying to wrap her mind around the horrible mystery of what was transpiring before us and between us. I wanted to fly away with her. Or at least to fly *her* away—as if she would leave me if she had the chance. I remembered asking her, when we were dating, if she would move to Iowa with me should I be offered the opportunity to attend graduate school there; we smiled, understanding that "yes" meant we would drop everything and go anywhere together. Now, her cry was the sound of a ruptured heart, whose ache I shared, the two of us alone in our separate beds in the dark. We cried together and managed to say goodnight.

Before the sun came up, I was wheeled to the room where I would spend the next three days. Somehow, I fell asleep.

• • •

Midmorning Wednesday, Dr. Eric Goren, a young attending internist, explained that until other specialists studied the results of the MRI, I was going to be treated as if I had a clot. An IV was already feeding a blood thinner into my left wrist, in hopes I wouldn't suffer another *attack*.

When my parents arrived from Lancaster, my dad did his best to wrap his head around all that had transpired since last night. He introduced himself to anyone who entered my room—no matter what color the scrubs—as not only my father and a doctor, but also an alum of Penn Medical School. He spared the doctors and nurses no questions. Their answers yielded little comfort or direction.

Dr. Goren, who insisted I call him Eric, returned to tell me it was not a clot causing the narrowing, but fibrosis—scarring. Yet there was a conundrum: veins didn't form scar tissue, at least not in the area where mine apparently had. He said he'd spoken to world-renowned vascular surgeon Dr. Ed Woo, among the most highly regarded doctors at Penn. "He's never seen this before," Eric said. "None of us have. But I'm talking to the smartest guys. I'm putting together the best possible team."

I was most comfortable reclined on the chair in the corner of my eleventh-floor room. Vana brought Nikitas to visit in the afternoon and again in the evening. After my parents left for the day, I wanted to call my friends, but talking wore me out. I kept my focus on the view, and on the progress I imagined in the sounds I heard beyond the curtain pulled closed behind me.

Beyond the window, lightning slashed the darkening sky.

• • •

On Thursday I got another CAT-scan, but there was nothing new. Everyone was puzzled. Eric said, "You understand, we're not used to this. We're used to getting answers."

Eric called in the chief of interventional radiology, Dr. Scott Trerotola, who explained to me that the only way to make a proper diagnosis was to do a biopsy—to somehow enter the chest and take a piece of the scar tissue. He described to me how he would have to enter through the vein and pierce the wall, then pull the fibrotic matter back through the vein.

"Okay." I nodded, picturing this.

"But it's too dangerous," he'd already decided. "The bleeding would be catastrophic."

So now what?

He seemed to know that he was my last hope—or that I believed he was—but neither of us said another word.

Vana and my parents stood nearby in mute dread, taking all of this in.

Before Eric left for the night, he confessed he didn't have a plan for me but didn't want to send me home. He'd take some heat for this—keeping me here day after day. Penn would have to eat the cost; insurance companies paid for progress being made, and progress was not being made. He told me I was the talk of the hospital, "a case study" destined to be the subject of a paper he or someone else would one day write. "You've stumped some very smart people who do not like to be stumped."

I imagined my story traveling like wildfire through the hallways. All I could hope now was that it would reach one doctor who would make it his mission to become the hero of my case study.

• • •

Friday, doctors filed in and out of my room in hopes of making a groundbreaking discovery. The rheumatologists examined my limbs. The thoracic surgeons contemplated their options. One suggested cutting me open from my throat to my sternum and across the ribs. But even with my chest wide open, they'd still need to get a piece of tissue from inside that confounding vein.

Then for several hours my room was quiet, and it seemed the investigation had ceased. I was afraid that the unsolved mystery had lost its allure to those who might solve it.

In the late afternoon the hallowed Dr. Ed Woo visited. I demonstrated how, when I bent over, blood flooded my veins and neck. He said, "Don't do that."

I grinned, trusting he knew we'd just acted out the old joke. *Patient says, "Doc, it hurts when I do this." Doctor says, "Don't do that."*

But he wasn't smiling. He said he was prepared to dismiss the need for a diagnosis. "Whatever caused the fibrosis is unknown. It happened. It's history." He said I would have to adjust to my new *idiopathic* condition, whose origins remained a mystery.

"Not bend over?" I asked.

"Not do a lot of things." He went on to explain how the venous system worked and *collateral veins* formed when obstructed blood found new pathways, not just deep in the body where they couldn't be observed, but also, he predicted, at the surface of the chest, where we would actually begin to see faint blue veins emerging. He said, "I think you're going to be okay."

I asked him to repeat this.

He said we'd do another CAT-scan in a month, and instructed me, in the meantime, to take life day by day.

• • •

The sun had set, and it was raining again. I sat in my hospital room, dazed and afraid. My sister, Sue, gathered her things and lingered by my side, where she'd spent most of the past few days. She was delaying her drive back to Lancaster, insisting on taking me home. I asked her to go ahead since there was no telling how much longer it would be until I was officially discharged. I stared out at the city, waiting for the nurse to bring my final papers.

I began to draft in my mind a letter I would email to my closest friends. I was trying to get the story in order, but for now my mind was a blur of unformed scenes, clipped conversations, disproven theories. *Dear Chris, John Bon, Mike, Alex, Lee, Ging, Dave, Jonathan, Matt, Fried, Dan, and Robin* . . . I was moved already by the realization that my list of addressees included twelve names—a testament to a life well lived. *How grateful I am to have you as my friends. I have thought of each of you, often, in the last few days, and though I didn't see you or speak with you, I felt your love, and it gave me hope—and the unquantifiable desire to be with you again soon . . .*

I reconsidered such sentimental expressions. *Just tell them what happened,* I instructed myself. I did not want to seem maudlin. But then, I wanted to tell them how I *felt.* This could be my last chance (*maudlin,* I thought, *but true*).

After nine o'clock I made my way outside, gym bag hiked over my shoulder as if I were going home after a workout. The night air was cool and wet. I could feel the seconds passing, all around me the slick patter of rainwater. The mysterious world of lights and life teemed with electricity. A taxi arrived at the curb, the spray from its tires whispering welcomingly to me.

While I was in the cab, Sue called from the road, and together we replayed what Dr. Woo had said about collateral veins, how blood backed up and found other routes, like traffic, and flow got back to normal.

Home, I stood in awe inside the screen door. Vana beamed from the kitchen. The house was still and calm, like the night in the wake of showers. Nikitas slept—a white cocoon aglow on the tiny blue monitor screen on the distant table. Everything in the room was spectacularly vivid: the paintings on the walls, the books on the shelves, the toys in the corner, the steaming plate on the coffee table—potatoes, zucchini, feta cheese fanned out beside slices of a French baguette. Vana sat by my side. She understood that what was here, right now, was exactly what this moment of my homecoming called for: the bare essence of the life we shared. She smiled, watching me eat what she had prepared. I savored each miraculous morsel. In a second, I saw this scene without me in it, an alternative reality—Vana alone here, with our son—playing like a phantom movie in my mind while my actual life went on. This sensation of the awareness of the seconds continued into the next day.

After breakfast, Vana and I took Nikitas to the playground, where he chuckled in the basket-seat swing that carried him from our gentle push, and I could hardly contain myself. There was nothing in the world beyond this moment. Nothing but the sound of my son's laughter, the touch of my wife's hand in mine. On the walk home, I told Vana it was about time I emailed my friends. But then I just stood there in the kitchen, watching her and Nikitas enjoying a snack. I questioned the relative value of writing an email now that every moment of my life had taken on a heightened sense of importance. Nikitas offered me a graham cracker. Vana gave me an understanding nod.

Upstairs, I settled onto my bed with my laptop. I asked my friends to bear with me as I recounted my experience of the last four days. As I began to write, I felt a welcome distance from the experience that had become my story. Telling it, I felt not triumphant, but simply alive, which today was a kind of triumph. *On Tuesday I was in my bedroom getting ready to go to the Phillies game, when I felt a sudden rush of blood to my head . . .*

When I looked up from my laptop, I was home again. And just like that, I felt I was walking on the edge of my life, with fear on one side—fear of those veins closing up, fear of what that fibrosis might be, fear of slipping away—and gratitude on the other side, for simply being alive.

3

BETHANY BEACH

We dared to stick to plans and head to the beach. We were taking the doctor's advice and trying to adjust to a new way of living. When I washed my hair and dried off with a towel, my head filled up like a fully expanded balloon. I sat on the floor to tie my shoes. I did my best to pretend that the genesis of my discomfort was, as I'd been told, *idiopathic*—the cause unexplainable, and the effect bound to improve. Meanwhile, I left Vana to do the heavy lifting and car-packing.

The town of Bethany Beach, Delaware, seemed like a movie set for a real-life fairy tale, especially at night when the world beyond the streetlamps, glowing storefronts, and quaint marquees sank into irrelevant darkness. At dawn, sunshine drenched the dozen or so square blocks of houses surrounding the commercial center and the short strip of boardwalk, where joggers leisurely loped along the dunes. After breakfast, my parents joined the community of unhurried exercisers, and, later, Vana followed suit, heading out in sneakers and shorts, pushing Nikitas in the stroller. At the end of the driveway, she hesitated and smiled welcomingly to me standing at the kitchen window above, double-checking to make sure I didn't want to join her. Of course I did. But at this point, even walking seemed to stress my system, stirring those ominous symptoms in my head and neck, so I was inclined to stay put. I waved to her and returned to my seat at the table, where my laptop had once again gone to sleep.

I was briefly soothed by the prospect of the morning routine—drinking coffee, working on my novel. At the table by the window, I riffled through note cards that outlined the thickening plot. But I couldn't stop thinking of Vana out there walking with Nikitas, the two of them alone together, a rehearsal of things to come, I feared. For a moment I bore down on the pages in my lap. But I was in no mood to write. Instead, I checked my email to discover encouraging words from my friends, who had read my letter. They had responded in turn, with love letters of their own. In the morning sunlight, I basked in them.

John Fried in Pittsburgh thought how lucky it was that this crisis had struck when it had, back in Philly, and not two weeks earlier during our trip to Berkeley Springs, West Virginia. "Who knows what the docs at that ER would have made of it. I'm just glad you're somewhere with the best people to look after you, if necessary."

Little did Fried know—but I would tell him when we talked later in the day—that after the CAT-scans and MRIs, and after the common, and a few uncommon diseases had been considered, a doctor had asked me, "Have you gone spelunking?" I shook my head—*as in cave-exploring?* The clinical interrogation had turned desperate, I thought. The doctors pressed on, asking if I'd gone hiking recently, in forests, or, yes, in caves, where I might have come into contact with a certain fungus that causes *fibrosing mediastinitis.* My stomach sank. *Oh God,* I thought. *Just last week. In West Virginia. With Fried.* This was it! Earlier, when asked if I had night sweats, I proclaimed that I was the king of night sweats; this summer I'd been drenching up to three T-shirts by the time I woke up for good. I'd been asked if my exercise routine had recently changed, and I recalled how, in the last month, the usual pushups had caused increased pressure in my head. And yet, there'd been no completely plausible theory—until I reported that last week I was in West Virginia, where I'd stayed with a writer friend in a rented house, and we'd worked on our novels-in-progress. But we were not aspiring Thoreaus, wandering in the woods. We'd spent our spare time playing tennis on nearby courts and grilling burgers on a raised deck. We *had* played horseshoes, I recalled. *Could this be the source of my potentially fatal ailment? Contaminated residue on a horseshoe? My skin brushing the diseased bark of a tree? An ankle grazing the wrong leaf?*

My parents returned from their walk. They finished a quiet conversation on the screened-in porch. They must have seen me in the kitchen, beyond the glare of the sliding glass door. They hugged, and my mother wiped her tears on my father's sleeve. They offered cheery hellos as they entered the house. Tonight, we would celebrate my mother's birthday, which fell each year during our week at the beach. She would eye the flaming candles, and we would all make the same wish.

When my father entered the kitchen where I sat, he studied my symptoms firsthand, unconvinced, as I was, that my condition was improving. Day after day we scrutinized the distended veins on my neck, measuring with our naked eyes their increasing size. I tried to quantify the relative venous "congestion" I felt when I stooped for a beach toy or pushed the stroller. When I rubbed suntan lotion on my shoulders, let alone when I dared to reach my shins and feet, blood flooded my head and those veins swelled. We wanted to believe that collateral veins were forming, increasing blood flow, while we dreaded the alternative possibility that the stenosis was worsening, that those veins were damming up in there. We told ourselves that the pressure I felt in my head was a good thing, that the stress was necessary to form collaterals—those miraculous bursting tributaries that would relieve my narrow veins and carry the blood from my head to my heart. Upstairs, my father sequestered himself in the one bedroom in the beach house where his laptop connected to the internet. Steadfast and devoted, he pressed on with his research.

My friend Chris from north Jersey called my cell phone. I went out to the deck, where the sun was shining. He assured me I'd be okay. "We'll be playing golf in our eighties," he told me. "We don't play *now*," I reminded him. The sound of his laughter relieved me. I was not yet forty-two, and I had just started a bucket list. "If I get through this, we aren't waiting till we're eighty," I told him. He happily agreed, as I pictured the two of us on some bright green fairway, in no hurry, following a white dot that vanished in the hazy daylight of summer.

I had not played golf in twenty years, for decades too driven by other ambitions to spend four precious hours strolling in vain toward a ball hellbent on straying from my intended path. And yet, it had always seemed to me a romantic game, a pursuit my ideal self might devote himself to, like yoga. In my twenties I'd devoted my summers instead to writing, limiting my exercise to the practical and efficient sessions I could squeeze in at the gym. Where was the boy who'd spent hours tossing a ball at a hoop or whacking a tennis ball at a wall at the park, trying to sharpen his dull skills at games he had no future in? But it was not too late, at least to dream, as I gazed toward the ocean and my friend's invitation crystallized in my mind like a calling to a new religion, which I was prepared to commit my life to.

Once again, I returned to the kitchen and my laptop. And once again I was drawn away from the work at hand, not unhappily, this time by a text from my teacher-friend Dave, asking how I was doing. I didn't tell him I had a sick feeling that my days at Penncrest High School this year were numbered.

After a shower my mother announced she was going to the supermarket, and before she was out the door asked if I had any special requests. Moments later my father followed, inviting me to accompany him with his laptop to the town park, where there was a strong Wi-Fi connection. Within minutes, the silence of the empty house made me feel hemmed-in. The laptop, the binder-clipped pages, the notecards wrapped in a rubber band all went into my backpack, and I was off to the nearby cafe for a change of scenery. I took it slow getting there, trying not to dwell on the discomfort in my neck and head.

At the cafe, a block from the center of town, I got my large coffee and lucked out with an available couch next to a table at the corner window. I set up shop, opening my laptop, arranging notecards in piles organized by chapter and scene, unedited pages in my lap, pen poised.

There was a knock at the cafe window behind me, and I turned to find Vana and Nikitas beaming and waving from the sidewalk outside, Mommy's sunglasses perched in her hair, baby in white beach hat velcroed at the chin. I smiled, relieved at the sight of them. *You have always known how to find me,* I thought. *And I have always loved being found by you.*

Vana circled the building and left the stroller on the porch. The bell on the doorknob jingled when they entered, their silhouettes haloed in sunlight pouring in behind them. I remembered Vana coming into view through the door of a restaurant where we'd agreed to meet on our first date a decade earlier, a setup arranged in the narthex of our hometown church by her mother and my brother-in-law, who hours later apologized to me and swore he'd only been joking around. I told him no apology necessary; I remembered the girl he was talking about, and I was going to call her right then and there. She was the most beautiful girl I had ever seen, having spotted her at church years earlier. Too young for me then, I believed; she was starting college when I had just graduated. But now the stars had aligned.

I set the untouched pages on the coffee table. My work was done here. For now. They joined me on the couch. Hugs. Kisses. "Hi, Daddy," Vana said. "Look, a pen." Nikitas reached for whatever he could get his hands on. "Daddy's book." Vana eyed my notecards, which to me appeared as pitiful stacks of countless untold chapters. "How's it going?" she asked. I shrugged. She rubbed my neck, her eyes faintly tearing. More kisses. Encouraging smiles. "It's going to be great," she reassured me. *Till death do us part,* I thought.

Hours later, walking on the beach with Vana, I felt the sand on the bottoms of my feet as a child might feel it for the first time, or as an old man might feel it, savoring what he knows might be the last time he enjoys a sensation. I felt the warmth and texture of my wife's hand, and of her face, as I remembered feeling it years ago when first falling in love. "In love"—this was the phrase I used to describe to her the feeling that had begun to consume my days, not only as I walked with her along the beach, but as I watched my son digging with a plastic shovel in the shade under the umbrella. I was "in love," *living* "in love," I tried to explain to her, understanding that no matter how long I lived, I wanted to go on living in this state of mind that seemed to shroud every sight I beheld in a kind of desperate glow of diminishing light.

At night we stood at the edge of the dark ocean. Under the sky's dim light, a grown boy and his father passed by us like ghosts of the future life I feared I wouldn't live. I wailed into Vana's hair, squeezing her with my whole being and howling my desperate longing to be alive to see that sight, the sight of my own son running. I swore in that moment I didn't care if I ended up paralyzed from head to toe, my life merely that of a witness to it all, peeking through a hole cut out for me to see the ones I loved living joyfully. Vana held me tight, absorbing my animal sounds that neither of us recognized.

• • •

The next week, I was eager to get back to school and my life as a teacher, hopeful that my work routine would somehow have a normalizing effect on my body. But then, on the first in-service day, after enduring the marching band's raucous welcome and the superintendent's inaugural address, I headed to my classroom, where I lamented the tasks I was unable to perform. My symptoms had worsened so much that I couldn't go on telling myself that all I needed to do was avoid bending over. I sank into my chair, surrounded by boxes and piles that required stress that my body couldn't bear.

And yet, for a long while, I sat at my desk and felt comforted by the familiar setting and by the daily routine ahead—the pre-rush-hour commute from the city to the suburbs, the programmed bells that signaled staff and students to start and stop, the rush of kids in the hallways, their restless vitality that gave me a charge. Each fall, time seemed to wind back to the beginning, as my students were once again eighteen, or they were about to be, and I felt one year better—not older. *How I have loved it here,* I thought, since that day in January 1995, when I'd first entered these hallways and understood I would leave law school for good and become a teacher, despite the secure future a career as a lawyer seemed to promise. *I would do it all over again,* I thought now, gazing at my classroom and recalling the countless students I'd taught and imagining the ones I could only hope to teach in the days to come. At the same time, I thought of my fellow teachers and the suffering we'd experienced together, especially during a surreal dark period years ago; all those kids fallen victim to unnatural death—suicides, car accidents, murders, drug overdoses—all those funerals we'd attended. I dreaded what grieving might be in store for my colleagues this year.

I pictured myself before a room full of students, as I took slow, easy breaths, hoping for enough stamina to make it through first period. Anxiety and sadness overwhelmed me, and I crossed the hall into the art classroom, where Dave promised to move every box, every desk, every chair, to do whatever I needed, no matter how much time it took. I didn't take for granted that I had a friend who was willing to work double-time to help me. "We'll get through this," Dave said as he escorted me back to my room and began to arrange tables, lug books, hang posters. Later, during an afternoon faculty meeting, I felt a wave of emotions swelling again, and this time Dave followed me out to the courtyard, where I collapsed on a trashcan, weeping, sensing by now that I was not going to be around this year. I told him, "I just want to live."

4

THE BEAR

Mike Fitz was home from Hawaii. He would spend the night at our place in Philly before heading to Lancaster, where we grew up. He knew the full story from the letter. When he arrived at our door, he conveyed his concern in a silent, strong embrace. Before long, Vana and I were bombarding him with questions—about fibrosing mediastinitis, collateral veins—feeling fortunate to have another doctor friend, who also happened to be a psychiatrist. We didn't disguise our desperation, taking full advantage of Mike's attention, and secretly expecting him to rescue us with his perfect combination of skills. He absorbed our restless expressions with stoic aplomb.

When Mike and I went next door to McCrossen's to drink beer and devour chicken wings, I recapped the full saga, hoping some unconsidered detail might inspire a crucial insight. I blitzed him with more questions, which the experts at Penn hadn't answered, but which I was expecting he might be able to. I was happy to provide a refresher course in the relevant anatomy, tracing with fingers on my neck and chest, where the jugular veins connected to the brachiocephalic veins, which connected to the superior vena cava . . .

He listened, shifting in his seat as I went on. Then suddenly, in the dark beery haze of the crowded barroom, Mike said, "I didn't come home for this," got up from the table, and turned for the bathroom.

I was stunned. At first I was thinking, *I didn't sign up for this either.* And then quickly I was filled with regret. When he returned, I apologized for putting him on the spot. He confessed that this was not the first time he'd felt bullied by me.

"Bullied?" Not a criticism I'd ever heard from anyone, let alone from my friend since sixth grade.

"I don't know the first thing about collateral veins," he said. "I'm a psychiatrist, for Christ's sake. You just keep pressing, and I don't have the answers you want from me."

I couldn't deny the accusations, that when I got swept up in my passions I expected him to match my intensity, in this case as I tried to piece together the puzzle or to find the narrative thread in a story he believed might be much simpler than I was making it out to be. "We just react to things differently," he said. "Especially when it comes to handling potential tragedies when the time has passed."

"This hasn't passed," I said. "No one knows what it is."

"Exactly," he said.

Wait and see, was Mike's philosophy, while I wanted to do everything I could to be prepared for what might come next.

"It was the same with the bear," I said.

He nodded. "You always gave that a lot more weight than I ever did."

"It was significant for me. It still is."

He grinned. "We were never in any danger."

"We didn't know that at the time. I'm still not so sure."

"Once the ranger said it was a black bear, for me there was no use in wasting another breath over it."

"We thought we were dead," I reminded him.

"But we weren't."

As we headed back to my house after midnight, our minds were reeling—at least mine was. I wasn't sure where Mike's head was at that point, but odds are it wasn't where mine was, set back twenty years earlier, out there in God's Country, fourteen miles deep into the wilderness of Yosemite National Park.

• • •

I'd wanted to turn back once we entered the meadow infested with mosquitoes. Mike and his brother-in-law, Darin, wanted to press on. I wanted to turn back when we passed the bearded man living in a tent. After we reached a clearing that Mike and Darin decided would be our campsite, I promptly crawled into the tent and slept in my boots and contact lenses, so convinced that we'd be seeing a bear that night, even after Darin reassured me that most campers who *want* to see a bear never get so lucky, that I had a better chance of getting struck by lightning, et cetera.

At midnight we shot up at the sound of a cracking branch. Mike and Darin had joined me after I fell asleep and now whispered, "What was that?" I said, "The bear." Not *a* bear. *The* bear. The one I knew would come tonight. We listened to the sounds outside our tent. The bear tore into the nylon tent bag, which Darin had tied to a tree twenty feet away and hoisted a dozen feet overhead—an impressive technique seasoned campers use to avoid attracting bears to their campsite. The bear tore into the bag's contents with ravenous delight. When the bear punctured the lids of our four tuna cans, with his nails or his teeth, the pops were like gun shots, spaced out several minutes apart. After the fourth shot, we braced ourselves.

There was a trickling creek on my side of the tent, and beyond the creek was a lake. The night was dark. The pale light of the moon reflected off rocks fifty feet away, visible beyond Darin's silhouette and the mesh screen that was the tent's zippered door. For hours, we listened intently. The bear would go silent for ten minutes, and then the sounds would return again and become closer and louder. We pictured him out there, investigating the campsite where Mike and Darin had made a fire. Darin offered to go out there and bang a pot to scare him off, but he didn't argue when Mike and I whispered no way. We're taking our chances and staying put, we insisted, understanding that this was an all-or-nothing gamble. If the bear came for us, we were finished.

When the bear finally approached, he pressed his body into the nylon wall on my side, to fit between the tent and the creek. "He's right here," I mouthed. "This is it." I had had all night to contemplate this event, and at this point I was incredibly calm. I was not going to die with bitterness or regret in my heart. My friend was visibly shaking with fear, so imminent was this threat. I was in a crouching position and holding his hand, trying to be encouraging. Not saying that it would be okay. I didn't know. Instead, I whispered, "If he comes at us, run." His hand was damp with sweat. His stare was hollow. It was pitch-black out there, but this is what I told them. "Don't fight. Just go." I didn't tell them what I had planned.

The bear turned at last to Darin's side and stopped. In the mesh panel the bear's head, inches away, was a dark shadow between the moonlight and us. His eyes glinted and teeth shone. His breathing was a rumbling thunder. I would be torn to bits. But maybe Mike would get away. I was as at peace with my plan, even as I was teeming with adrenaline. I had never faced anything like this. Nothing so terrifying. Yet I was about to give this bear a run for his money.

The three of us stared straight back at the bear, who was looking inside the tent at three sets of eyes staring back at him. Somehow we kept our cool, all three of us stock-still. Seconds passed, maybe ten, during which we sent that bear a message.

He was just standing on all fours. His head was more than a foot wide. There were six inches of black nothing between his shining eyes. He breathed big heavy breaths and decided finally he'd had enough of us. He'd kept us in suspense for four hours. We understood once he turned and trotted and jumped over those rocks that he was gone for good. In an hour the sun would be rising and we would be able to leave this place.

"Holy shit." We could breathe. Even laugh. The moment the sunrise provided enough light for us to see the world outside the tent, we crawled out, examined with horror and relief the tuna cans and other ravaged possessions, and packed up what we could. As we marched toward the trail, I kept my eyes peeled for movements beyond the nearby ridge, where minutes earlier I'd spotted a mound of rocks I was sure was the bear's den.

The walk back was quiet and quick. Hours long but quick, nonetheless. Mike and Darin hustled to keep up with me. We came to a crossroads. A wide stream. A river really but the current was slow. The trail went along the water. We mapped it out in our minds and estimated we could save ourselves an hour if we could somehow cross that river. I didn't deliberate for long, leading the charge, knee-high in ice-cold water, pushing straight through to the other side.

We changed our clothes by the trunks of our cars. We snapped pictures as if to document our survival. Mike and I had been planning to travel farther west, or south, to LA or San Diego, before heading back east, but not anymore. Darin reported the experience we'd had to a park ranger, who neither shook his head nor raised his eyebrows, unimpressed by the tale. He said he couldn't say for sure what would or could have happened, or whether we'd just been spared from sure death, but he speculated that it had likely been a black bear. Not a killer brown bear. Not a bear looking to eat three dudes in a tent.

This possibility, of a black bear, as opposed to a known killer, never diminished the significance of the event for me. I had in those long four hours faced death and resigned myself to it, determined to save my friend by sacrificing myself. I had recited in my mind Dylan Thomas's poem, *"Do not go gentle into that good night. Rage, rage, against the dying of the light."* I thought of that night, of those crucial hours, as my finest moment. You don't know how you're going to act in such a situation, but I'd found myself ready to fight the bear to death for long enough for the others to flee—as if there weren't a chance in hell I would suffer a failure of nerve or be torn to shreds in an instant. Of course, the bear might have caught up with them if I weren't enough to satisfy his appetite. But I wouldn't have known any better by then.

The truth was that the ranger had only been guessing. It wasn't impossible that the bear had had it in him to take us all out. I could never say for sure. You just can't know these things. You're left with your memories, which are always reshaping themselves, becoming more or less significant in ways that your evolving life requires.

• • •

After the beer and wings at McCrossen's, Mike and I hovered in the dark outside my house, not yet ready to call it a night. "I'm afraid," I said. In an instant Mike appeared shocked back to his wits, wide-eyed, as if recalling the purpose of his visit. "I'm *afraid*," I repeated, understanding now, as Mike did, that the beer and talk of anatomy had driven us both off-track, away from the fear we shared.

The next morning, we headed to Starbucks on the corner. I confessed I'd been thinking again about that night twenty years ago. He humored me. We made a more explicit connection. The woods. The bear. Confronting potential death together, but never really knowing for sure what risks we faced. I apologized again for missing it last night, for failing to see how hard this must be for him, and how relentless I could be, how my clinical questions and talk of medical mysteries must feel like badgering, making him feel worthless and helpless as a doctor and a friend, no less helpless than I felt.

He shook his head no, as if I had it all wrong. "Let's not forget what a complete asshole I was last night," he said. "I'm a psychiatrist, for Christ's sake." He grinned.

We walked back from Starbucks, coffees in hand.

5

LABOR DAY WEEKEND

The plan had been to return to the beach, but when Vana suggested we stay home to be close to the hospital, I didn't argue. By now, I was puffing up on the right side of my neck, feeling a soreness in the muscle that rose from my clavicle to my ear.

I was as disappointed as my brother, John, who looked forward to our annual tradition of shutting up the beach house for the season. At sunset on Monday, the two of us would go bike-riding on the quiet Bethany Beach streets. Then we'd feast on hard-shell crabs at Mike's on Route 1, cracking away on the picnic table covered with thick brown paper stained with butter and beer. Walking back to the house, we'd pretend to be townies, relieved to be rid of the vacationers, before getting into our cars and driving back to Philadelphia.

Instead, I was home, understanding that Vana's caution pointed toward something inevitable that we could not drive away from. In our townhouse I was reading an email from my friend Dan Peterson, who had aced the high-school chemistry class we'd taken together, and who was now an internist with a group of physicians in nearby Mount Airy. It turned out that, since reading my letter, he'd begun to make it his part-time job to find a diagnosis. He didn't want to bombard me with the research he'd done. He said feel free to call or even come straight to the office.

I called him immediately and headed to Mount Airy to join him for lunch. We met at his favorite tavern in town. He didn't like the look of the puffy flesh above my clavicle. He believed fluid was building up, a sign that the body was trying to heal itself. He suggested we keep a close eye on the area until my scheduled CAT-scan.

· · ·

Given my description over the phone, my father believed I might have strained a muscle. But when my parents visited from Lancaster, he changed his opinion. The swelling had made its way around the base of my neck. Something was going on in there, and it wasn't collateral veins forming.

Dan and my dad traded theories over the phone. In the late afternoon my dad called Dr. Woo, who was on vacation at the Jersey Shore. He told my dad to trust his instincts and, if my symptoms worsened, to send me to the emergency room. When no one was looking, I packed my gym bag. I packed the book I was reading. A baseball for good luck. When my dad got off the phone, Vana and my parents turned to see me standing in the doorway, ready to go.

In the ER my dad and I didn't have to wait long before my name was called. After an EKG I was whisked back to a room of my own in the emergency wing. I got the CAT-scan we'd hoped I wouldn't need for another month. It showed similar obstruction, but nothing revelatory. I was scheduled for an MRI, but it was Labor Day weekend and service was slow.

A young doctor explained that both she and the attending radiologist, who had already examined the CAT-scan, were confident the obstruction was a clot. "Just a clot," she said. Clots passed, she explained to me, or at least they could be treated. I was relieved to hear this diagnosis. *A clot. A clog.* I pictured Liquid Drano clearing the pipes.

The purpose of the MRI was to confirm that it was just a clot. But there were only two MRI machines available because there were so few technicians on duty. (Everyone was at the shore!) Another young doctor explained to me that the priority patients were emergency cases, people with giant tumors on their spines, for example. Fortunately, I was not an emergency case.

After being admitted to my upstairs room, I was assured, once again, by the first young doctor that I had a clot. She and everyone thought I had a clot, she repeated. When she said this one too many times, I began to believe that what I had was definitely *not* a clot. She reminded me that the MRI would confirm it was just a clot. She told me to be prepared to be awakened in the middle of the night to be taken downstairs for the MRI. She offered an apologetic smile, as if quality sleep were my main concern and the MRI, a nuisance.

• • •

I was disappointed to wake up fully rested Sunday morning, having never been awakened for an MRI. The weekend dragged on.

In the afternoon my cell phone rang. I picked up, despite the unfamiliar number. A man said that shooting for the TV commercial would begin next week. I believed he had the wrong number until he said, "From Sears." And then I remembered the recent scene as if it were from a lifetime ago—the two women stopping me on the sidewalk, asking if I would answer a few questions for the camera. The man had my bio right there, he said, and the video, which looked good, he added. He said I should wear my own clothes to the shoot and they'd provide the Sears attire when I got there. Finally, I told him something unexpected had come up. I was sorry I wouldn't be able to do it. He said it was no problem, and the call came to a quick close. I realized his list was long. The campaign would go on without me. Sears would survive another day.

Staring out the window at the city, I contemplated the ever-spinning world. The sun was burning bright. I pictured my brother on the beach, mourning the end of summer, dreading what fall might bring. School would start on Tuesday. I'd called my boss. I didn't know when I'd be back, I said. Or *if.* "Don't worry about things here," were my principal's encouraging words. Lessons would be taught, he meant. The school would survive.

On the sill sat the half-read novel I wouldn't bother opening because novel-reading wasn't of any interest to me, any more than novel-*writing* was. The novel I wouldn't crack open was John Irving's *A Widow for One Year,* whose title's irony I wouldn't recognize until I continued reading it months later while in bed next to Vana. I couldn't bring myself to write a blog or keep a journal, or even to take notes so that I might one day document these experiences. The moments were far too precious to do anything other than subsume myself in them entirely. Gazing at the trees and sky over low-lying buildings in West Philly, I flipped in my hands the baseball I'd brought from home.

· · ·

Vana and I held hands and watched the cool blue sky turning gray. I was grateful to her mother, who was home taking care of Nikitas, giving us time to be alone. Vana had brought fresh T-shirts and boxer shorts. She'd brought me leftovers from dinner, her mom's tomato chicken and fresh-cut french fries cooked in olive oil. My appetite was restored. Vana told me what funny things Nikitas had said today, and how he seemed to be on the brink of walking on his own, how he'd guided himself along the edge of the coffee table and then to the ottoman, where he'd held himself up in front of the TV and danced to the music of the farm-animal video.

"I'm sorry you're going through this," she said.

"I'm sorry *you're* going through this," I said.

We smiled and kissed and stared into each other's eyes. It was as if we were summoning up all the moments we'd been together and, when the tears started again, the moments we'd yet to be together.

I remembered, on the brink of a breakup a decade earlier, her saying, "I just want to *be* with you," as if imploring me to comprehend the simplicity of the matter. I, the restless fool, convinced myself that this sentimental expression defined the essence of our differences, rationalizing that she was content just to *be* together, while I was itching to *do* more together—or *not* together, as it were. At last, I came around and took the long view, realizing, after four years of dating, that *being* together was what couples did most of the time, between whatever "doings" they did.

So here we were, just being together, and it was all I wanted, though I was saddened by the thought that this was not what she'd had in mind—nor was I *who* she'd had in mind, this diminished version of me. I was nonetheless grateful just to be together as we were at this moment, not to be doing anything in particular.

That is, until we agreed that I needed a shower. She understood this meant *her giving me* a shower, as I was hindered by not only the IV pole but the severe discomfort that accompanied any twisting and bending. The IV pole had a reserve battery pack, so we unplugged the long cord, and she helped me maneuver myself and my machinery into the bathroom. She undressed me and guided me into the tub. The shower head was portable, so I tried to help, but even spraying myself triggered instant congestion of my head and neck. Vana took over. I stood tethered to the IV pole on wheels, parked at the tub's edge. She drenched me. She lathered the washcloth. She washed my hair and body. "Want to get in?" I teased. "Yes," she played along. "My big strong man." We smiled ruefully, imagining a different version of this scene. She rinsed me. She dried me. She guided me back to my chair.

I was standing in a towel, about to ask for fresh clothes from the bag on the windowsill, as she rifled through her large purse, which I assumed contained the few items she needed to spend the night here. Then keys jangled in her hand. When she looked up, I must have appeared more puzzled than disappointed, so convinced had I been that she would be staying with me tonight, so crucial every moment had become, at least in my eyes—sitting, eating, talking, bathing—each of these activities a kind of sacred ritual.

"I'm not leaving yet," she assured me, and set down her purse. She handed me a fresh T-shirt and boxers. "I have to get back. There's the bedtime routine, then the morning routine. It's too much for my mom." She was digging into her purse again, head bowed, for something precious. "I need to get his lunch ready. I need to make sure he gets to bed."

"That's why your mom is there, so you can be here with me. It's only eight o'clock."

She shook her head. "Damn it. Where's the—" She plucked out the parking-garage ticket. Her shoulders sank with relief. "I haven't been sleeping at all, and there's no way I'm going to get a good night's sleep on this chair." She gestured to the chair I spent my days in, then looked out the window, across the city, in the direction of our home. "My mom is worried about me. She says I'm spending too much time at the hospital. I need to take care of myself so I can take care of . . ."

I couldn't believe what I was hearing.

"Worried about *you? I'm dying!*" I snapped.

She didn't look at me.

"Don't you realize what's going on here?" I felt unhinged. "Doesn't your mother realize—? Aren't you telling her what's happening? You can't possibly be telling her! No one would say something like that—*you're spending too much time at the hospital!*"

"Stop yelling!" She glanced at me, her eyes cool, though wet with tears. "Your face is purple."

I couldn't calm myself. My crying turned to sobbing. "You're supposed to be here with me. You're my wife. I'm going to die."

"Stop," she said softly. "You need to relax."

She meant it, for my sake. I caught my breath. I repeated, for good measure, "You're supposed to be with me." I felt separated from the world, not just the world outside these walls, but the world outside my skin.

"Don't blame my mom," Vana whispered. She wiped her tears. "I haven't slept. Do you understand? I have to go. I have to take care of our son."

She took the T-shirt and boxers from my hands. I sat down and she slipped the shirt over my head, jimmied the shorts up my legs. I took deep breaths. I wiped my tears. I stood. We hugged. We were crying together. But I was thinking, *I'm alone.* And then, *We are all alone.* I believed she was thinking the same thing, and yet I couldn't help blaming her for protecting herself, or her mother for protecting her daughter.

"I just want to be with you," I said.

"I want to be with you, too," she said. "And you're right, I *should* be here. Tomorrow night, I promise."

"Okay," I said, though I recognized a voice of duty, not passion. Her face was pale and expressionless in the shadowy fluorescent light by the curtain hiding my bed. I could now see why her mother was concerned for her daughter's health, in spite, or because, of how grave mine might be. Of course, Vana must return to Nikitas, whom she could care for, feeling that the love she provided him would make a difference.

"Get some sleep." She pulled the curtain aside and guided me into bed.

• • •

When my dad arrived Monday morning, he was surprised to learn that the MRI had never been canceled, only delayed by the two young doctors who remained convinced I had a clot. By now, my father had been in contact with Dr. Woo, who explained that it had been he and Dr. Trerotola who'd stopped the MRI. I was amazed to learn that on Saturday night Dr. Woo had left his family in the middle of dinner at a local restaurant to examine my CAT-scan on the computer back at his beach house. He then called Dr. Trerotola, who was also on vacation with his family. They determined that what I had was not a clot, but something else that was constricting the blood flow through the veins that led to my heart. They'd concluded that what I needed was not an MRI but a venogram, which I would get first thing Tuesday morning, when the hospital kicked back into action.

By Monday evening, my dad lost patience with the two young doctors still defending the merits of the MRI—and of the theory that I had a clot. He snapped, "Who is in charge here? Who is taking care of my son?" He asked them when they'd graduated from medical school, and the one said, "A couple years ago." My dad said, "So, 2009?" I watched all of this from my bed, my eyes widening with surprise. The other one said sharply, "The question shouldn't be how old we are, but how good we are at what we do." My dad said, "Well, we'll see."

I was slightly embarrassed to see my father scolding these young doctors, who turned silent in the wake of his insinuation. But mostly I wanted to high-five him. I had not once in my life seen or heard him speak to another person—let alone another doctor—so curtly. For over thirty years he'd guided young residents, and no one looked upon the representatives of his beloved profession with higher regard than he did. I saw now with thrilling anticipation that my father was prepared to pull out all the stops to save me. It was as if his whole career had led him to this ultimate and unfortunate challenge.

Later, alone, I stared out the window at the black sky. The night's dim spots of light, from the streets to the stars, shone as if through holes poked through heavy paper. My eyes rested on the shadowy shapes of the city, and it occurred to me just how alone I'd feel anywhere else but Philadelphia, this city filled with faceless strangers who seemed, even now from this distance, somehow familiar to me. This place had become my home. I loved this city as a child loved his bedroom, comfortably surrounded by his collection of sacred objects, his taped- and tacked-up pictures, reflecting the identity he had begun to imagine for himself.

By now the staff had angled my bed almost at ninety degrees to keep my head up and my blood flowing down. I existed precariously at the mercy of the universe's mysterious forces and its dependable forces, such as gravity. I no longer needed to bend over to feel the blood backing up in my head and neck. Pumping through the IV that accompanied me day and night, heparin kept my blood anti-coagulated. At last, tomorrow's plan was a firm one: Dr. Trerotola would be performing the venogram first thing in the morning. It wasn't a clot we were dealing with here. I didn't need an MRI to tell me this. The stars in the sky told me—what few stars were visible tonight.

6

THE HELMET

Ordinarily I didn't have trouble sleeping, but tonight was a different story. I called up memories of the summer to ease my anxious mind. I thought of Nikitas and me sitting at our favorite fountain, Vana and me lying on the beach. These memories became like waking dreams I hoped would become my actual dreams.

I pictured the three of us walking to the playground the morning after I got home from the hospital just over a week ago. It was a day we wanted to believe marked a new beginning, since I was home again, though without a diagnosis and floating in a state of tangled hope and dread. From the sidewalk Nikitas pointed to the playground, and we took the shortcut through the baseball field. Out of the stroller and into the basket-seat swing he went, giddy with anticipation. Vana and I shared in his delight—his protective helmet off for good now. The memory was another welcome dream, of a seemingly idyllic time, its pleasantness tinged only with the recognition that whatever hope we'd had that day had dwindled.

Six months earlier, in March, Nikitas had been diagnosed with ITP—*idiopathic thrombocytopenic purpura*—a blood condition characterized by insufficient platelets, which are crucial for healing and clotting. His pediatrician had noticed a constellation of tiny purple bruises, *petechiae*, on his belly and back. For protection from internal bleeding, he had to wear a helmet, a chin-strapped, brown foam job resembling those worn by yesteryear's football players. One of his parents had to be with him always. For three months, Vana and I alternated days off from work, an arrangement that took me out of the classroom and Vana out of the office at the university where she'd just been promoted to associate dean.

Before Nikitas's illness, my plan for the summer had been to finish writing the novel I'd been working on. I'd been looking forward to waking up early, taking him to daycare, and returning home to write until it was time to pick him up after five o'clock. For the last seventeen years as a high-school English teacher, I had allowed myself this luxury—ten weeks to live the life of the full-time writer.

Plans changed. Summer came, and his platelet number continued to plummet. Now he would be staying home with me every day. The healthy platelet range is 150-450. Nikitas's level lingered at 20, having dropped from 35 when he was diagnosed. If the number dropped below 7, a platelet transfusion would be necessary, though it wouldn't provide a cure. If the blood did not normalize on its own in six months, his condition was likely to be permanent.

My days began when Nikitas woke up at six. We went downstairs and played on the padded mats while Vana slept. He handed me books and crawled onto my lap, where he turned the pages. We started with *Hey, Wake Up!*, my favorite. *"Morning snack is here for you, milk and cookies and broccoli stew. Eww. For the bunny, not for you."* He drank his bottle of milk. I fed him breakfast in his highchair, where he was safe from contusions. I took off his helmet, which he called his "hat." I took off my Phillies hat. We wore our hats when we played. These were circumstances I would not have chosen, but they had provided an opportunity I was now grateful for.

When Vana left for work at eight-thirty, Nikitas and I went outside for the first of our two walks. We made pit stops at the swing sets near the ball fields and the Art Museum. We returned home for lunch. He wouldn't fall asleep in his crib, so by two o'clock we were back outside again, this time for the longer walk, when he slept for more than two hours. When the stroller stopped, the nap stopped, so I wore running sneakers and kept moving.

I listened to audio books, feeling productive while pushing the stroller. I figured that if I can't write, I can at least read—or be read to. I devoured massive volumes. I stored up ideas inspired by the books I was reading, hoping to find time to write myself. As the summer went on, I varied the routine, taking detours to different parks and playgrounds. Nikitas and I scoured the dirt for sticks and stones. When he fell, I checked his body for bruises. We sat on the benches near the Rodin Museum and expanded our vocabulary. "Tree." "Bird." "Sculpture." "The Thinker." I drank iced coffee from Starbucks to keep me charged. Nikitas played with the straw. He reached for the cup of ice when I was finished drinking. I thought of how, whenever I got hiccups, Vana recited, "Give me your hiccups, give me your hiccups," with ritualistic devotion until the hiccups relented. When the time came, she expected the favor to be returned; I always obliged, with the usual eye-rolling. Now I found myself pleading with Nikitas, *Give me your. . .* not really believing I could influence fate with my thoughts. Nikitas smiled and shook the cup of ice to make music.

This was the best summer of my life, I decided, despite the challenges Nikitas had presented. I found myself in no hurry to finish writing my novel. By July, I had him napping in his crib. By August, I had him falling asleep at night on his own. Once he was going to bed without much fuss, Vana agreed to take on bedtime duties, freeing me up for an hour. I said an early goodnight to Nikitas and with my laptop headed to Starbucks, where I made slow but satisfying progress on the novel. Vana bathed Nikitas and gave him a bottle. By eight, they were reading *Goodnight Moon.* He fell asleep within minutes after his helmet hit the bed sheet.

I returned minutes after Vana called me home. We had about an hour together before we began to doze. We ate our late dinner on the big chair, our trays on the ottoman. We watched the Phillies in their glorious season. Vana became a genuine baseball fan. I agreed to watch reality shows about rich housewives. This was the life we'd created together. We did not take for granted the time we were sharing, attuned to the synchronicity of our three lives so intertwined. There were moments when we didn't think about Nikitas's condition, or the danger his helmet was protecting him from, despite the bruises that bloomed almost instantly after even the softest bumps and falls. We'd been told that the body had the capacity to heal itself. We were counting on this healing to occur by September so that we could all return to our normal lives.

In August his platelet level dropped to 7. We handled him like a large overripe plum.

Then, on my second day in the hospital, a nurse called with the latest results, by chance dialing my cell phone instead of Vana's. She was calling from right next door at the Children's Hospital. The platelet count had jumped over a hundred points, she said, to 134. Sitting in my chair at the window of my hospital room, I sobbed tears of joy for my son, who'd never known his health was in jeopardy. Just like that, he was back to normal, his body having performed its own healing miracle.

At the playground that first morning I was home from the hospital, Vana and I stood together, in confused awe, hoping for another such twist of fate. Our son beamed from the swing, returning to us.

7

DOOMSDAY

When I woke from pleasant dreams Tuesday morning, a white lab-coat apparition appeared at my bedside. Dr. Trerotola shook my hand and assured me that the procedure would go well today. Then he explained that, because of his booked schedule, there was no way he could do the procedure himself. My heart sank. But he promised to be in the room when the pictures were taken and evaluated. I suggested we postpone the procedure until he could do it himself. He said there was no time to delay.

Vana arrived, and the two of us—I on a gurney and she by my side holding my hand at the edge of the mattress—entered the hallway and began the day's unfathomable journey. This was another in a series of long rides to some faraway room where we hoped to make progress, down hallways and elevators, pushed by a kindly orderly who greeted along the way his cheerful coworkers, nurses, and doctors. All the days I'd been here, these people had made the place seem to me like a vigorous organism, a body magnificently thriving, despite its afflictions, or because of them, compelled by the drive to heal itself, healthy cells and sick cells together in the common goal of wellness.

I was wheeled into the center of a large cold room. Vana and I kissed goodbye, and I watched her exit through the stainless steel doors. Two nurses circled my bed, making preparations. An old Jon Secada CD played, and I was half-tempted to request a change in the music, or at least to crack a joke about this soundtrack, which was weirdly incongruous with the event at hand—or it was too painfully relevant. *Mornings alone . . . Give me a reason . . .* Instead, I made a game of it, testing my tolerance for these sad lyrics of longing and loss, wondering if these nurses had considered the potential effect that deliberately heartbreaking ballads might have on a patient poised at the edge of the abyss. *It'd never be the same if you're not here . . .* I couldn't help thinking that Jon Secada had been selected not by accident, but with the best intentions. Someone believed that *Just another day without you . . .* helped create a relaxing atmosphere.

Dr. Stavropoulos put me at ease, despite the music. He was very tall and handsome, like an actor who might play such a dashing doctor on a soap opera, soothing a patient like me at a time like this. It was not hard to believe—or at least to pretend—that, in the world Dr. Stavropoulos inhabited, nothing went wrong. I was sedated and drifted off into a kind of wakeful oblivion. I was shrouded in music-free white noise, stainless steel sparkling on the periphery of my consciousness. I was aware of the needle entering near my neck, dye entering my bloodstream. In the world of the others in the room, time passed as they did their work. In my world, time stood still.

And then awake and conscious, I was staring up at a glowing triptych at least two feet high and twice as wide. Magnified in sharply contrasting black and white was an area of my internal anatomy that I instantly recognized as freakishly abnormal, my eyes drawn to the vertical black line that looked like a hot dog with a toothpick stuck on top. The toothpick formed the base of a Y. The arms of the Y, I could guess, were the brachiocephalic veins, which I knew branched toward the jugular veins on each side of the neck. But what this toothpick was, I didn't understand.

Beside me stood a group of doctors, all in white coats: Dr. Trerotola,

Dr. Stavropoulos, Dr. Woo, and a gentle blue-eyed fourth man I had not yet met. Vana had arrived, and she was smiling warmly at me.

They had all been waiting for me to return to them, and I was back now. Dr. Trerotola explained that what we were looking at on the screen was the place where the X-ray picked up the dye injected into the bloodstream during the venogram. Anything black indicated blood flow. Anything that was not blood flow appeared as white light. The hotdog was the SVC—the superior vena cava—the main vein entering the heart. The toothpick, he gravely said, indicated the amount of blood flowing into my SVC from the brachiocephalic veins. To be clear, the toothpick should be as big as the hotdog. The negative space around the toothpick—just white, borderless light—was where the unidentifiable obstruction was, the mysterious fibrosis we wouldn't yet call a mass or a tumor because these words suggested malignancy, and this obstruction did not appear to be malignant; it was too symmetrical, they all agreed, too smooth, like a perfect doughnut, unlike malignant tumors, which are asymmetrical, jagged, and ugly. We were all staring at the obstruction on the screen with a kind of perverse admiration. "Just look at that toothpick." "Never seen anything like it." "We just don't know what this is . . ." So weirdly, perfectly cylindrical, just like the doughnut surrounding it, the light between, constricting the blood flow and expanding outward, and outward, just as I felt myself beginning to drift, beyond the borders of the screen, and into infinite brightness.

I returned to the voices, all four men agreeing once again that the first option, to do a biopsy, was too risky. Dr. Trerotola had not changed his thinking since his first visit, weeks earlier; doing a biopsy could lead to internal bleeding. "I could kill you," he reiterated. What's more, even if he managed to procure with a long needle some bit of the mass, whatever it was, the pathologists could find it to be no more than unidentifiable fibrosis; or the mass, or tumor, if that's what it was, could be disturbed by the needle and break into pieces that spread into the bloodstream. The second option was to remain in an observation mode. This was not really an option, since I had what appeared to be between 5 percent and 10 percent blood flow through the toothpick into my SVC, and no one knew how long the vein might remain even so marginally open. The third and final option was surgery, but no one knew what the surgical strategy would be, much less the prognosis.

· · ·

In the late afternoon, Dr. Woo visited my room. Though my breathing remained unrestricted, it seemed I was being strangled from the inside a little more so each hour, the backed-up blood pressing at my eyes and throat. He reiterated the three options: observation, biopsy, surgery. No hope for collateral veins, he said, because there was simply no time for them to form. Biopsy, too dangerous. Other interventions would mean a lifetime, however brief, of disability, symptoms, and irreversible disfigurement, what with the clotting, stenting, ballooning, and the inevitable disintegration of the irreparable veins.

I was sitting next to Vana on my hospital bed, my parents in chairs at the opposite wall, getting the straight truth from Dr. Woo, who told us—after all the research and the CAT-scans and the venogram, after the department chiefs and specialists had examined me and all reached the same conclusion—there was nothing left that they could do. Beyond the large corner window, the city of Philadelphia looked sad and magnificent in the rain, the red and white lights sparkling in the darkening day.

The end would not be pleasant, Dr. Woo was saying. It would not be a good life for the brief time I might survive. My father nodded. He had no more questions. Dr. Woo sat with us in silence, which supplied all the answers. I understood that I was going to die soon. I was here with my wife and parents, who would bury me. I wanted to save them from such grief. I hugged and kissed Vana. We cried together on the bed. I imagined myself in the coming days, maybe weeks, propped up in bed like a bloated specimen, transformed by one vain procedure after another. "I'm sorry," Dr. Woo said, and left the room.

I hugged Vana as a young widow I could not save from grief. We were poised at the edge of an ocean of sadness. I tried to offer her what comfort I could, as years of agony loomed like a dark force rising on the horizon.

My parents made their way toward the rain-spattered windows. My mother sat and looked out at the gray afternoon. My father stood behind her, the two of them alone in their own measureless sorrow. They sobbed quietly. I had known for one year how it felt to love a son; I could not imagine how it felt, after four decades, to witness his death. I rose and, draped in my white cotton gown, made my way toward them. I hugged my mom and said I'm sorry. She was strong, or numb, holding herself together. I hugged my dad. I stroked his silvering hair, something I'd never done before. He cried on my shoulder, something he'd never done before. "I'm sorry, son," he said. For the life you will miss out on, he meant, and for missing out on your son's life. "I'm sorry, Dad." For having to bury your son, I meant. He set his pale blue eyes on me and said, "Tomorrow more research. More research." It was an expression of pitiable desperation. It was also an expression of infinite and illogical hope. He did not have to explain the contradiction to me. "We go on," he said.

My father appeared dazed by the sight of me. I could see him after I was gone, weeks or months after the funeral, chin up, eyes downcast, gait slowed, my mother, by his side, appearing stoic, no tears left. I imagined Vana clutching Nikitas at her chest, trying to explain something she couldn't understand; my friends, huddled together in dimly lit restaurant booths, puzzling over my absence. I felt myself already slipping away, and yet, somehow, I felt more alive than ever. I wanted them all to know that I felt pure gratitude for the life I'd lived. I was amazed by these feelings. Amazed to realize that what mattered, and all that had ever mattered, was right here before me, in the present moment. To understand that this was not the pit, but the pinnacle.

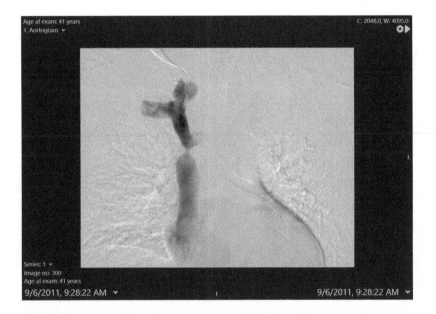

8

HAIL MARY

The attending internist on duty today entered the room to find my parents, Vana, and me huddling hopelessly together. She hesitated at the doorway. When our eyes met, she offered a quiet smile. I could read her expression. She was determined to keep pushing back against the vague forces of inertia pressing in on my shrinking world. I had told her how I fantasized about sitting with a radiologist, right there in front of all the films, comparing the images that had accumulated and asking the questions I'd developed, somehow to reconcile once and for all the apparent contradictions between the earliest readings and theories from my visit weeks ago, and those from the past week.

Now she informed us that Dr. Miller, the top chest radiologist, was willing to speak with us, indeed, to discuss the films, right there while we all looked at them together. We rose to our feet, some vague hope emerging, if only at the prospect of comprehending the dreadful fact of my untreatable syndrome. We were moving forward, or at least moving, resisting the deadly pressure of resignation.

On our way to the elevator, we saw Dr. Trerotola walking toward us. He'd just come from Dr. Miller, who was "a true wizard," he said, as he gladly did an about-face and walked with us back to the basement of the hospital, where the radiologists study their films. I felt like a president getting the executive treatment, being transported in Elevator One. Dr. Trerotola prepared us for what we were about to see, describing what he'd just seen himself—pictures that confirmed our grim outlook.

Low-ceilinged and carpeted in navy blue, the lab had the look of a think tank, a secret meeting place for backroom strategists. Just inside the entrance, Dr. Miller sat before three large screens featuring black-and-white images of my superior vena cava. Beyond Dr. Miller, other radiologists sat silently before their respective private screens, several of them peering in our direction, curious about a family who had entered this sacred space to get a firsthand look.

I felt both cursed and blessed, sitting shoulder to shoulder with Dr. Miller, Dr. Trerotola standing beside us, my family behind us, all our eyes transfixed. Mouse at his fingertips, Dr. Miller escorted us into the three-dimensional virtual world of my chest, our eyes traveling down a roller-coaster vein that arrived suddenly at a massive white doughnut with a small dark hole. He wound around to give us a view from every angle. In speechless awe, I was gazing at the future cause of my death. No autopsy would provide a better view. I sat at the edge of my seat. I began to describe, out loud, with a preternatural understanding, what it was that we were all looking at, explaining with strange satisfaction how it all made sense to me now, finally, reconciling the various theories and explanations I'd gathered since my first visit three weeks earlier. I could see now why some doctors had concluded from the earliest scans that the obstruction was less in the SVC than in the brachiocephalic veins—that is, less in the *trunk* of the Y than in the *branches*. I could see now in all its mortal glory how the obstruction was one perfectly cylindrical mass that rose from the SVC and into the brachiocephalic veins. This was the living proof that I couldn't survive much longer with such limited flow.

Dr. Miller kept his eyes on the screen as he talked. "What this obstruction is, exactly, is still cause for much debate. Fibrosing mediastinitis, maybe. But as we've said, this fibrosis appears to be *inside* the vein wall. Which means it *can't* be fibrosing mediastinitis." The contradiction was a familiar dead end. He shook his head.

"Even if it's benign," Dr. Trerotola began, "biopsy could prove disastrous, since matter could disperse into the body."

Dr. Miller set his eyes on me. "At this point what matters is not a diagnosis." He looked at Vana and my parents, then back at the bewildering image on the screen. "To be frank, this tumor, or fibrosis, or whatever you want to call it, *needs to come out. Period.* Whether it's malignant or not." He looked up at Dr. Trerotola, who nodded, the two of them, and all of us together, at the crossroads. "Now this is a question for Dr. Pochettino."

I thought, *Who is this Dr. Pochettino?*

I shook Dr. Miller's hand and thanked him for this privileged glimpse. On our way out I asked, "How many times have you done this before—sat here like this with a patient?"

He grinned. "You're it."

• • •

We had been cautioned that Dr. Pochettino was extremely busy, in surgery all day, so we should not expect to see him anytime soon— certainly not tonight, but maybe not tomorrow either. He needed time to look at the films and to form his own outlook.

Around 6:30 p.m., my parents were out in the hallway, updating my sister on the phone, and into my room walked a gentle blue-eyed man in blue scrubs, white coat, and running sneakers. Dr. Pochettino, I presumed. And then I realized that he was the fourth doctor who had been standing by my bedside after the venogram. I stood to greet him. We shook hands and sat. He spoke with an elegant, slight-Italian accent. Vana and I were instantly at ease, confident in the presence of this calm, pleasant-faced man, who summed up our grim options once again. Only this time the doctor concluded by saying something much more. "Or, what I will do is go in and take it all out and reconstruct the SVC with a material that I have been using for several years and with much success."

Vana and I couldn't believe our ears. This was the Hail Mary pass, I realized, the last-second play that was not in the playbook. And I was game. Vana rushed to the hallway and returned with my parents, who sat with us and listened patiently. Vana asked him to repeat what he'd told us. We were astonished and bewildered all at once, overwhelmed with joy and gratitude, tainted by a distant fear.

Vana asked him to explain exactly how the surgery would go. He explained that he would be using a material called CorMatrix, a post-organic composite made primarily of pig intestine, which he had used extensively to patch hearts and lungs. It worked like a scaffolding that my own cells would grow onto like ivy onto lattice. My cells would *endotheliolize*, taking over the graft, which in months would be resorbed into the body with no side effects. Vana pressed him for more details. He explained that he had done innumerable heart and lung transplants, but only two SVC resections, neither of which had been as complicated as this one.

Vana was apoplectic. He answered the question she couldn't seem to articulate, or didn't dare to ask. "I plan to restore your husband to normal health. He will be in critical care for two or three days after surgery and then another week in the hospital. He will be home in a week to ten days and then back to work in perhaps three months." He smiled. We remained speechless. It all seemed too fantastic, that I might live, let alone return to normal life. He concluded, "We can do the surgery tomorrow or Friday. I don't do surgery on Thursdays. Thursdays I make my rounds and see my patients."

And just like that we were talking about not *if* but *when*.

I looked at Vana and at my parents, then back at Dr. Pochettino, who awaited my reply.

Hours later, my parents, Vana, and I would sit in this same dark corner of my room, contemplating the next step. They would deliberate about options and second opinions. They would consider flying me to the Cleveland or Mayo Clinic. I would tell them that everything we'd been through in the past few weeks had led us to this moment. They would not argue when I told them we were not leaving this hospital or this one man who had looked me in the eye and said he could do this.

"I would not wait until Monday," Dr. Pochettino added.

"Friday," I said.

He smiled. I nodded. Vana and my parents looked on in amazement at the surgeon and the patient who had entered suddenly and separately into their precious pact.

Not tomorrow. Friday. I would need at least a day to recover something I'd lost, or nearly lost, completely.

"So there's hope?" I asked, still in awe.

He said, "There is always hope."

I mirrored his smile.

We stood and shook hands. I gave him a hug, which he modestly returned.

"I will visit you on Thursday," he said, "just to check in. But we're on for Friday."

9

BIG BROTHER

In his dark Italian suit, my brother appeared, a force to be reckoned with—wherever he showed up—especially in my hospital room first thing Wednesday morning. In a few minutes he would be heading to his office a dozen blocks away. Right now, John fielded another in a series of calls on his cell phone, stepping into the shadows behind the curtain by my bed; he signaled to me with a finger, as if he were holding me up, though I had settled into my chair by the window, poised for a full day of visitations and long-distance phone conversations with friends. John and I had been chitchatting about the surgeon's plans and the cutting-edge material made of pig intestine that would be replacing my SVC. John would be here first thing Friday morning, he promised; he said he'd always appreciated my being there with his wife before his own surgery nearly twenty years ago.

"Sorry about that," he said, returning. "Anyway, now I get to return the favor. I'll stay with Vana as long as I can, at least until Mom and Dad get here. Unfortunately, I've got a deposition that morning. What time's the surgery?" He glanced at the vibrating phone in his hand. "Damn," he whispered, "sorry."

I smiled as he ducked behind the curtain.

I'd always felt empowered in John's presence. As little brother, eight years younger, I would watch in awe as John would throw a baseball straight up into the sky, beyond the highest leaves, and I'd wait for it, a shadowy dot returning to earth and landing in my glove. That's how it was growing up. I followed his lead. He was the picture of success, the essence of cool. When the time came, he'd take me along on dates with his girlfriend. In college, at Franklin & Marshall, not far from our childhood home, he'd take me to his fraternity house, where his other brothers called him "Greek," and me "Little Greek." As a young lawyer, he'd host me in Philly, take me to the office, where I imagined working one day. Even as my distinct identity began to take shape—in high school, after he was gone from home, and at Bucknell, a few hours north, as I studied literature and art—my instinct, at least for the big decisions, was to do what he did.

Now, I imagined that the doctors and nurses were stepping up their game, seeing that I had *this guy* on my team, even if they didn't know what he did for a living. The truth was that John had represented clients in more than a few medical-malpractice cases involving doctors at Penn. He recalled a recent cocktail party in the suburbs where he was chatting with a surgeon whose wife warned her husband, only somewhat in jest, not to show his cards to the lawyer representing the plaintiff. John is well-liked, seen as understated and charming, not just by his clients but, I imagine, even by the defendants he might be suing for damages. He was sure that by now my doctors had identified him—for better or worse, we joked. I was comforted by the belief that the Hippocratic Oath would keep their minds unclouded, regardless of my connections.

"Sorry." John was back again. He leaned against the wall by the large window, checking the messages springing up on his phone. "I have to get going. Mom and Dad on their way?"

"Later," I said. "Dad's got some meeting Friday he has to prepare for. He called this morning to tell me."

"Wait—Friday? The day of your surgery? What meeting?"

I shrugged. "He said he doesn't want to cancel it if he doesn't have to. He'll be here when I wake up, he said."

John's eyebrows shot up and his head sank. "No," he groaned.

"It's fine," I said. "He said he's in charge of this thing that took forever to put together."

John pressed his palm to his mouth as if to muzzle himself. I knew what was coming; I could sense him making the connection, reaching reluctantly into the past. He took a deep breath then let it spill into the room. "You know he did the same thing on the day of *my* surgery."

I shook my head. "This isn't the same. He's been with me every waking second for weeks. I've been his full-time job."

John gave me an expectant look.

I conveniently ignored the inevitable question, in no mood to contest John's vague theory about our father's absence or to explain, again, my simple one.

"All right," John said quietly. "I gotta go, unfortunately."

"Don't say anything to Dad," I said. "It really is fine."

"I'm not saying anything."

I returned John's gentle handshake.

"Besides, I'm going to be under anesthesia," I tacked on, trying in vain to make my case.

John grinned wryly, as if sparing me the truth—some deep point I was not quite grasping or not yet willing to admit.

"I'll try to stop by later," he said. "Otherwise I'll see you tomorrow."

After John left, I thought about how I'd always felt secure in the knowledge that my father and brother had my back; and now they understood, as I did, that for the first time in our lives, there was nothing more they could do to help me. I'd always enjoyed the luxury of carving out my own path, all the while trusting that, come hell or high water, there would be a backup plan. After guiding me in the directions of their careers—toward medicine, toward law—my father and brother supported me when they saw my true interests taking hold. When I found myself halfway through Temple Law School, my brother's alma mater, reading novels and writing short stories instead of lugging around textbooks and studying for my exams, John encouraged my decision to drop out, advice my dad hesitantly supported, concerned I wouldn't "make it" doing whatever else I might end up doing.

This week, the jokes my friends made, considering my unusually— if not mortally—afflicted superior vena cava, had been, "Jeez, Jim, why do you always have to be so original?" "Yeah, couldn't you have just gotten a massive tumor?" "Or had a heart attack?" I had resorted once again to memories of my brother, as an example of grace under pressure, recalling vividly that period twenty years earlier when his daughter, facing death, needed another new liver and, when a second donor didn't emerge, John didn't hesitate to offer half of his. I remembered my sister-in-law, petrified, not only at the prospect of losing both her daughter *and* her husband, but at the thought that she hadn't given John a way out of this dilemma, that he'd been pressured into performing this potentially fatal, or at least futile, act. I assured her that there was no stopping him, that I'd never seen anyone so certain of his path in life, however altered it seemed now.

My dad had attempted to relieve the pressure on John, telling him in the hallway of the hospital, as if conveying a dark secret, "It would be okay, you know, if you didn't do this." I'd stood silently there, awaiting my brother's reply. The implications were obvious. This was, in John's eyes, confusing medical advice from the one doctor whose opinion was hard to ignore. My brother, appearing stunned but vaguely grateful, said, "She's my daughter. You'd do the same for your child." My dad said, "I'm not so sure."

Two decades later, my brother still hadn't shaken this puzzling exchange, periodically mentioning it to me, perhaps anticipating my different interpretation. I had been alone with my sister-in-law on the morning of my niece's and brother's surgery, until shortly before the operation, when my parents arrived. And now, coincidentally— or, *not* coincidentally, as my brother believed—my father had already announced to me that he would not be at the hospital when I went in for surgery this Friday, but would arrive shortly after the procedure had been completed. He would attend a previously scheduled meeting in Lancaster, before driving with my mother to Philadelphia. "I'll be there when you wake up," he'd assured me, vaguely apologetic about the crucial appointment he said he really shouldn't miss if he didn't have to.

Forty-eight hours from now, Vana would spend the morning alone with her fears, while my brother, determined to keep her company while I was in surgery, would get stuck for hours on 76 East, driving into the city, cursing the traffic backed up because of an accident.

My belief has always been that twenty years ago our dad meant to let John off the hook, to take the weight of responsibility off his shoulders, seeing that his son was prepared to give not just half his liver, but his life, to save his daughter. I believe he meant to express admiration for John's bravery and selflessness, and it was a confession of sorts to admit that he really wasn't sure what he'd do if the roles were reversed, which isn't to say that he wouldn't have done the same thing. I believe he would have. But, until you're in such a dire situation, you don't really know how you're going to react. You're thrust into the fire, and you just react. You retreat to safer ground, or you head into the flames. I don't believe my father was speaking to my brother as a doctor, cool and clinical, offering medical advice. I don't believe it was insensitivity that explains his blunt admission, or even his delayed arrival on the day of surgery. I believe that, for those few hours, when there was nothing more he could do to help, he retreated to safer ground. I believe he was a father afraid for his son—then, for John, as he was now, for me.

10

COMMUNION

Wednesday afternoon I sat in my reclining chair at the window facing West Philly. With each deep breath, I sought connection to the world within this building and to the one beyond the glass that separated me from it. I gazed out over a verdant canopy of leaves covering uncountable city blocks. I thought of the air the leaves supplied with the oxygen I breathed. I imagined, down below, students and workers crisscrossing on the sidewalks and in the grass, off to the classroom and to the office, briefcases and steaming cups in hand. Overhead, cotton-white clouds floated in a field of perfect blue, all I saw before me aglow in the sunshine, bound in a teeming flow of energy I tried to feel a part of.

Outside the window to my left was the contrasting industrial image of the roof of the adjacent building, a stony field speckled with metal-box compressors, fans, and vents, which I recognized as the ports that drew in, filtered, and circulated the air I pulled into my lungs. I was in awe of the universe's unfathomable interactions that made life possible.

Lining the windowsill were my framed photographs—Nikitas and me at the fountain, Vana beaming as a new mother—and a folder including the printout of the venogram, which today I would display for visitors trying to grasp the full weight of my condition, and the surgeon's imminent challenge. In my hand was the baseball I flipped and turned, the seams winding infinitely under my fingertips, the worn-horsehide aroma musty as an old garage.

Friends visited. We sat in the well-lit corner by the windows. We talked optimistically of my looming surgery, while right now inside my chest a nearly occluded SVC, the most crucial vein, supplied my heart with only a small percentage of what it normally provided. Heparin dripped from the pole tucked into the corner behind my chair, the clear liquid doing its work of altering the blood's makeup so that it could make its way through that shrinking toothpick opening without clotting.

I called the friends who couldn't make it in person. John Bon in California pointed out that this experience was testing every philosophical idea we'd ever sat around pontificating about; he meant that this experience had tested not just me, but him, the observing friend who must prepare for the possibility of his own great loss. He recited Joseph Campbell, romantic adages on courage that over the decades we'd pretended to live our lives by. "The goal is to live with godlike composure on the full rush of energy, like Dionysus riding the leopard, without being torn to pieces . . . As you go the way of life, you will see a great chasm. Jump. It is not as wide as you think." He said, "It's not just an idea now. You're doing it." I felt a charge that would sustain me into the OR.

My dad had called an old friend from medical school, a psychiatrist, Dr. Peter Bloom, who visited. It was not long before I forgot his profession, thinking of him as a kindred spirit. He was a skilled soother of souls. We found our common ground in books. I told him I'd been thinking about Zorba the Greek, whose zest for life seemed to increase in the face of calamity. I recognized the paradox; the more love and joy Zorba dares to experience, the more pain and loss he must endure. That is the passion, not unlike Kazantzakis's re-imagined Christ, whose suffering seems intensified in the torn soul of a man who triumphs over the temptations of the flesh. I confessed to Peter that, for reasons I understood were tangled up in such passions, I couldn't bear to see my son this week. Vana and I had painfully agreed that at this point it was best she not bring him to the hospital while I sat here reminiscing and hoping, resisting and accepting all at once my desire to return home. Such was the struggle I tried to welcome, the price to pay for a life filled with love. I tried joking with Peter, quoting Zorba. "Am I not a man? . . . wife, children, house, the full catastrophe."

Peter told me about *Full Catastrophe Living*, by Jon Kabat-Zinn, a master of mindful meditation; then he taught me a mantra for the difficult moments he anticipated I'd be having often between now and Friday, and, God willing, paradoxically, even more often *after* Friday. "Every day, in every way, I'm getting better and better." Since my physical condition would only worsen without treatment, the irony of the quote pointed toward its higher purpose, of psychic well-being. Peter explained that the quote comes from the French psychologist Emile Coue, who promoted optimistic autosuggestion. The words already rang true as I breathed in, reciting, along with Peter, "Every day in every way," and breathed out, "I'm getting better and better."

· · ·

My friend John Pritchard, a Methodist minister, popped in, apologizing for interrupting, and offering to come back later, just as Peter prepared to leave. When Peter stood, I insisted he stay. This was a meeting of the minds, to be sure. I believed that the peace I sought lay at the intersection of traditions embodied by these discrete thinkers—the spiritual realism that had countless times inspired me in my minister friend, the graceful touch that disguised the clinical intentions of my new doctor friend.

The three of us were chatting when my hometown priest called. Peter and John talked quietly with each other while Father Alex told me that word had traveled to Lancaster, where many people were praying for me. My attention was torn, as I didn't want to miss whatever insights Peter and John might arrive at together while I was distracted. Here was a convergence of powerful energies, the voice of my childhood church on the line, while before me sat these two men whose distinctive perspectives, brought together here, no doubt held potential truths I couldn't bear to miss out on for a second. Over the phone, Father Alex recited a prayer of healing. I closed my eyes and began to cry. John and Peter had gone quiet. The air was imbued with a benevolent force I felt giving me strength. "We love you," Father Alex said. "I love you, too," I said, and by "you" I meant whomever he meant by "we." I believed he was speaking for thousands. When I opened my eyes, John and Peter offered me their encouraging expressions.

We sat in silence. Tears fell onto my frozen smile.

After Peter and John left, I recited, in my solitude, my new mantra, breathing in, "Every day, in every way," breathing out, "I'm getting better and better . . ."

• • •

My last visitor Wednesday was Father Christ, from the nearby suburban church we'd recently begun to attend. When he read a prayer for healing, I felt my body flood with energy that rose through me and left me calm. He gave me Communion; he dabbed holy unction onto my forehead and hands. He shook his head at my incredible story and assured me he would visit again after surgery.

Once I was alone, my mind drifted inevitably to images of Vana with Nikitas across town, having a snack or an afternoon nap, unless she left him at daycare down the street so that she could come visit me here or buy groceries or cook dinner or go for a walk or catch up on the phone with her boss, who continued to reassure her that the university would survive without her for at least a little while longer—or so that she could do whatever else people do when their spouses are poised at the brink of the abyss and they feel torn in opposite directions, drawn to higher ground, their instincts at odds.

I sought solace in memories—of our first date, in Manayunk, lunch, followed by strolling in and out of the town's motley shops, whose wares made no difference to us but served as props to our banter that might prove endless as we wound our way through a furniture warehouse displaying couches we sampled, in rooms we pretended could be our own, crossing our legs and chatting and laughing and soaking in brief silences, as if rehearsing for some future house, before retiring to a coffee shop, at sundown, and wrapping up, for now, our great debate about art and movies and how to distinguish "best" from "favorite," and I agreed to rewatch *The English Patient* and she agreed to watch Scorsese and Coppola, "But first, how's Friday?" I asked, "Dinner in the city?" and she nodded, yes, "Sounds good," and then she said, "Oh, you mean *this* Friday?" and I laughed, *of course,* and in the pause that followed while sitting in her car I wanted to kiss her, naturally, but I didn't feel hurried—I felt transported—thinking of Friday, and every day after that, and so I shook her hand and she giggled at that.

Five years later we were married, and five years after that we had Nikitas, whose birth needed to be induced, and so on the night before his arrival we watched our two favorite movies, *Sideways* and *Lost In Translation*, stories that featured youngish middle-aged characters struggling to say goodbye to their seemingly idyllic pasts, when all that existed and all that seemed to lie ahead was pure potential and inevitable long-lasting happiness. The next day, labor was long and difficult. Vana managed to resist epidural relief until the eleventh hour, when contractions, as forecast by the administering nurses, produced toe-curling pain. She was left nonetheless to deal with a torn pelvic muscle and weeks on crutches and months after that the emergence of those tiny purple bruises on her baby's body and the need for that helmet to protect him from bleeding, and months after that her husband's freakish breakdown.

Now, as the hours swiftly passed in the dark hospital room, I was surprised by my own surging sorrow. I was suddenly sobbing so uncontrollably that I woke my roommate, a tender-voiced man recovering from lung surgery. Hearing me struggling to keep it together on the other side of the curtain, he called out from his bed, "Nurse! Nurse!" then got himself up and out into the hallway and hollered—with his one lung—"My man needs help in here!"

• • •

My first visitor Thursday was Father Alex, who'd driven the hour and a half from Lancaster, surprising me. When he spread out onto the deep windowsill his tiny black briefcase containing a spoon and small bottle of wine, I didn't mention Father Christ's visit the day before, happy to repeat the ritual. He read prayers and blessings. I welcomed Communion for the second time in two days. When he left, I felt ready for what was next.

My teacher friend Dave dropped in with cards and well-wishes from my colleagues at school. The superintendent called and wished me well. I felt inspired by my growing audience of encouragers, whose generous energy I hungrily absorbed.

As promised, Dr. Pochettino visited, wearing the familiar blue scrubs that matched his eyes. I arose from my recliner to greet him. He asked, "Are you ready?" Mirroring his grin, I answered, "I'm ready," and added, "Are *you* ready?" We shook hands, partners in a great undertaking.

Evening approached, and I was once again surrounded by family. We sat together for hours, with no thought of being elsewhere, until it was time to say goodnight.

Vana stayed.

After eleven I made the last of the phone calls to my friends. For reasons I realized only when Lee was at last on the line, I had delayed this final call. I was not prepared for his cheery optimism, his beery confidence. Nor was I prepared for one of his timely spot-on insights, like the time he said that Vana was *"too good* for you," which at first I stupidly interpreted as the obvious insult it seems to be on its face, before I understood that he was cleverly observing how much she and I had in common, for better and for worse, he explained, pointing out just how "perfect," or *too good,* a match we were, and warning how being such a match brought unique challenges, different from those faced by couples who were attracted to their opposites.

"Jimmy!" Lee greeted me. I heard a football game on the TV in the background, the same game my roommate was watching beyond the white curtain. I explained the plan for tomorrow. He heard me choking up. "You sound terrified," he said, and I felt accused, a bitter emotion I could barely track, countering his buoyant tone. He was going on, "I've been thinking, and I realized, why not Jim Zervanos?" He repeated this, "Why not Jim Zervanos?" I felt pushed to defend myself. I never believed I should be exempt! He pressed, *"Why not Jim Zervanos?"* and I began to understand that he was not directing the question at me, or at least he was not expecting a satisfying answer. He filled the silence between my stuttering non-replies, the two of us a tangle of words, and then his voice softened, and we were quiet.

"It's okay," I said, surprised at my own tender expression, content to let his question go unanswered, to let this last goodbye feel incomplete. "I should go to bed."

The parting was quick. I felt unbalanced. Vana asked if everything was all right.

Minutes later the phone rang. Another old college friend said, "I just talked to Lee. He's been keeping us all in the loop with emails and phone calls. I wanted you to know we're all praying for you."

And just like that, balance was restored. I smiled, teary-eyed, imagining Lee, my devoted, passionate friend, pacing furiously in his New York City apartment, phone at his ear, spreading the word, ripples of love expanding outward into the glittering night.

I felt an irreversible momentum as I settled under covers. Since this morning my roommate had been greeting my friends and family as they filed in and out. Tonight, I welcomed the vital sounds of the game from beyond the curtain. "Goodnight," I called, pleased to think that my old friend had my back. "All right, my man," he reassured me.

Vana pushed the reclining chair next to the bed. Then she climbed in and lay snug next to me.

11

AWAKE

First thing in the morning and we were off into the bright hallway, on my miracle mile. Vana escorted me on my gurney to the preparation room, a vast white space where we met the young anesthesiologist resident who explained how things would go in just a few minutes.

I'd already been told that my wife would be there when I woke up, and that first I'd awake with the breathing tube, and they'd quickly get me back to sleep; then later they'd wake me up for good. I'd been instructed to rate the level of pain from one to ten when I awoke the second time. I'd been told this ahead of time, I understood, because it would be hard to communicate with a patient who was delirious with pain and anesthesia. The hope was that the pain itself would remind me of these instructions.

Vana stood with me now in the waiting area, various sections of it cordoned off with curtains outside the operating room. She elegantly disguised her fears. I was grateful to behold her poise and beauty here, to absorb one last dose of prayerful energy from one who loved me; we held hands, feeling each other's touch, cheek to cheek, absorbing each other's warmth. Unreasonably, I had no doubt that I would be seeing her again in a few hours. I attributed this irrational confidence to the distracting power of love, which I had welcomed hungrily for two days, and to the cool optimism of the surgeon who had taken it upon himself to save my life.

Before long I was wheeled into the OR, a cold fluorescent white room where I was hoisted onto a narrow table. I stared up into bright lights. The attending anesthesiologist, a middle-aged man with a peppery beard, kept the mood upbeat with his smile and good cheer. He said we'd get started in a moment, and then the mask was on my face and in seconds I was gone, gone for five hours to a place of no thought or memory, despite the electric saw that split the sternum, the machine that pumped the heart, the hands that snipped and stitched with exquisite precision—these magnificent feats accomplished for my sake while I existed in a merciful blankness that might prove eternal.

As promised, I awoke with a tube in my mouth, or *that's what this must be,* I thought, this most unnatural intrusion that wound through my throat and into the center of my being. The moment was one of surreal shock, the awareness of life striking my consciousness at the same instant I feared death by suffocation. This staggering misery lasted only seconds, during which time I was a thrashing non-person, unhinged with confusion. I gagged and choked and tried to scream, and then I couldn't comprehend what was happening before I was gone again.

As promised, I awoke the second time and Vana was there. I felt her touch, I heard her soothing voice, and yet, instantaneously, I was screaming, "Ten! Pain!" somehow recalling those pre-game instructions. It appeared that she was hearing me, as I called out to her, as instructed, and so *Why isn't anyone doing anything?* "Ten! Pain! *God!* Ten! *Pain!*"

Vana gently turned to whoever else was out there and said, "I think he's saying something."

How was this possible? She couldn't hear my words! Somewhere from beyond the agony, my sense of humor returned, along with the full recognition now that I was alive and I was feeling the pain that was promised upon my awakening, and I was howling at the absurd, hilarious, beautiful world, "Ten! *Ahhh, Goddammit! Ten!*" Vana's ear was at my mouth, as the scream I meant to be blood-curdling was coming out as a whisper that needed translation.

She told the doctors and nurses, "Ten, he's saying. His pain is a ten, he means."

• • •

I was fully awake now, sitting up. Magically—or thanks to morphine—the pain was gone, and there in the doorway, standing at the line they were not permitted to cross, were my mom, dad, and sister. And, just over their shoulders stood Dr. Peter Bloom, whose warm and welcome presence was hardly necessary to remind me of the words he'd put into my head. Before he could prompt me, I said loud enough for Vana and all of them to hear, "I'm getting better and better." They smiled, and then I heard the chuckles I was hoping for.

I'd made it through to the other side. I felt alive and grateful, the fruit of some miracle growing inside my chest, which pounded and pulsed with a dull throbbing force I welcomed.

For two days I recovered in critical care, in the same room I'd awakened in. The catheter, which unbeknownst to me had been doing the work of emptying my bladder, was removed. And now I couldn't urinate. When a drop threatened, my whole body clenched, resisted, so intense was the pain. When a drop got through, I collapsed on my bed in muscle-melting agony. Simply to *will* the urine out of me, despite the torment I anticipated, was impossible but necessary, I was told. My nurse helped me to my feet. She stood at my one side, Vana at the other. A woman on each arm, providing physical and emotional support, as I was about to embark toward this great milestone. A sucker for any audience, I was determined to do this. I tried to relax, to purge the pain into the urinal the nurse held for me at my thighs. They waited. We all watched as I released a drop, *ahhh, God,* no. I clenched up, and then a sputtery stream. "Yes?" I gasped. *No way. Can't do it.* We all watched passively, me too, as if progress might happen down there with help from some separate, masochistic plane of my consciousness. I was a hopeful observer, as were my two encouragers. I told the nurse that this was quite a way to get to know each other, the three of us hanging out like this. She'd heard all this before. She laughed sympathetically, Vana nervously. The laughter transported me beyond the numbing pain, and soon I was emptied out.

Later my nurse bathed me with soapy cloths as I sat up in bed. She had two patients to attend to; two was the standard, she told me, and we would keep her busy all night. I was amazed to be the focus of such generous, tender attention. The care she provided seemed uniquely extraordinary, profoundly personal, and I was humbled by the thought that she had devoted her life to giving this same treatment to countless other people, night after night, day after day. She spent the whole night with me, or so it seemed, not gone for long, leaving and returning, as she divided her time between me and her other patient. The night felt like weeks, the pain in my chest literally paralyzing, the two of us awake in a dim blue room that transported me to a kind of black hole, cut off from the life I'd once known.

In the morning she came to help me out of bed. I couldn't fathom that they had me moving to the chair beside my bed already. I was told that movement was the way toward healing, and so from bed to chair I went. My breastbone felt about to crack. At night, back to the bed. These short trips marked the start of the long recovery. The dressing was removed from my chest. My nurse swabbed the wound. Protruding from my skin under my rib cage were three clear tubes, each the width of a finger, that served to drain the surgical site during the operation, and apparently post-op as well. The tubes extended from my body and hung off the edge of the bed, out of view, emptying into a clear plastic jug. On the second day, with help from an assistant, my nurse placed me on my back. She gripped the first tube and on a count of three, with clenched jaw, yanked it like a stuck plug from its socket. Black stitching popped from the gash— as planned, she told me. She did the same to the second tube. She removed the strings, though one bit of thread dangled, tangled, stuck despite her tugging. It would come out in its own time, she told me. The body would naturally reject foreign matter as the wound healed and sealed up. The third tube would stay in for another week.

My brother-in-law, Niko, visited and gave me a watch that was too nice to wear in the CCU—a gorgeous thing with blue hands and a black leather band. I imagined wearing it in the classroom. Metaphors of time abounded in my head. I put on the watch and then removed it for safekeeping. The gift made me happy. Its uselessness to me now enhanced its beauty.

• • •

The next day I was shipped off to the cardiac wing, where all the patients, most of them three or four decades older, shared the same clavicle-to-sternum scar visible through the gaps in their gowns. They shuffled up and down the hallway, men and women, arm in arm with a physical therapist, one hand gripping an IV pole, a bag of heparin hanging from a hook. In a few days I would be joining them. For now, I sat snugly in the chair next to the bed, the pain in my chest creeping in like the tide. I pressed the pain button, and a narcotic wave rolled through my body. I'd been encouraged to keep the pain at bay, to use my pain button, so that I could work on restoring my breathing to normal. Bigger breaths meant increased pain—but no pain, no gain, my nurse told me. My expanding lungs pressed against my ribs and strained my wound. I pictured the steel coil holding my sternum together stretching at the seam.

Dr. Pochettino visited. He described the black muck he'd removed along with most of my SVC and two nearby lymph nodes he cut out just to play it safe, though he believed the black muck was benign. *The black muck*—he mentioned it as if an afterthought, though the obstruction had confounded us for weeks. It was all out now, he said. That's what mattered. He'd planned on cutting out two centimeters of the SVC, but once he got in there he kept cutting until the vein was clear. Six centimeters, as much as he could, he said, right down to the azygous vein, which met the SVC at ninety degrees, leaving about a third of the original SVC. He described the Y-shaped graft he'd sculpted with sheets of CorMatrix, which he'd rolled into vein-like tubes and attached to the remaining segments of my SVC and brachiocephalic veins. I pictured him securing the Y's base to the tree-trunk stump of my SVC and fastening the Y's arms to the severed branches of my brachiocephalic veins above. The CorMatrix sheets were six-centimeter squares, he explained, and he'd needed all six centimeters. He grinned, acknowledging a bit of good fortune—good thing he hadn't cut the graft down to two centimeters before realizing he needed all of it. *Good thing.*

I looked forward to going home. I hadn't seen my son in almost two weeks. I had no desire to read or write. I sat in my chair and recited the mantra Peter had given me. "Every day, in every way..." I discovered Angry Birds on my iPhone. I had never been a player of video games, even as a kid when friends were drawn to their dark basements to play Space Invaders on Atari, and to the arcade to play Pac-Man. I'd always preferred baseball, even when it meant going solo, chucking a ball against a wall or hitting a ball off a tee. But here I was now with Zen-like focus, pulling the birds back on the big slingshot and watching them sail toward the green pigs. *I'm getting better and better.*

I maintained a low-grade fever. I sweated through my T-shirt, boxers, and sheets three times a night. The young nurses responded to my calls, at midnight, at 3 a.m., at 6 a.m. They changed my sheets. They detached my IV tube and helped me change my soaked shirt.

As the week went on, we all awaited the pathology report, pretending that the diagnosis of that black muck was purely academic, an afterthought, of no consequence, and why not, after what appeared to have been an incredibly successful surgery, which had resulted in the replacement of almost my entire SVC with a graft made of pig intestine and the removal of an unimpressive substance the surgeon seemed confident was benign.

12

THE DIAGNOSIS

I would be going home on schedule, just a week after surgery. It was amazing to think that I would be back to my normal life in three months, as Dr. Pochettino had predicted. They started me on Coumadin, an anti-coagulant pill, to replace the heparin still dripping from the IV pole that had become like a third arm in the past month. Once the transition was successful, I'd be on my way—but not before we got the results of the pathology report.

On Wednesday afternoon my friend Jonathan Rubin was visiting when a young doctor in a white lab coat entered the room. Red-haired and slight of frame, he introduced himself as Dr. Dan Landsburg, a hematologist fellow. "Dan," he said. We shook hands. The preliminary pathology report was back, he announced, and, pressing his eyes on me, asked if it was an okay time to talk—okay to talk with Jonathan in the room, he meant. I understood that this question was a bad omen. I nodded, glad that Jonathan was with me to hear whatever unwelcome news Dan was about to impart. He took a seat across from us, wasting no time. I realized that such unfortunate visits were among the young fellow's errands.

"So, you've got lymphoma."

The word *lymphoma* seemed both devastating and meaningless.

My mind sought a reference point, some context for cancer in my life, a way to begin to formulate what this information meant for me. Jonathan and I sat silently, absorbing the diagnosis, which seemed incongruous with everything that had happened till now. And yet it also felt like the most natural progression of events—*of course the black muck wasn't benign!*—another blow that sent me against the ropes. I felt myself floating, falling. The floor seemed a long way down.

Dan couldn't yet identify the type of lymphoma, couldn't say whether it was Hodgkin's or non-Hodgkin's, not that either category would make any difference to me. Nowadays, he explained, we avoided these broad categories, whose names had taken on false or misleading connotations. Instead, we used the very specific names of the kinds of lymphoma, of which there were over forty identifiable types with drastically varying prognoses. "We just don't know what type yours is yet," he said. We would know in a few days. The slides had been studied, but more time was necessary for further testing.

When Dan left, I recognized in Jonathan's teary-eyed expression my own sadness and fear, mixed with a resilience that together we'd built up over the past weeks. One day soon we would try to articulate this feeling we shared, this numbness that had become strangely familiar. We should not be so comfortable with this new information. We had developed a taste for the absurd. *What kind of lymphoma is it? The deadly kind? The curable kind? The undiagnosable kind?* Perhaps mine was a kind they'd never seen before, a kind they'd need a new name for. I imagined the slides with my cancer cells in a top-secret envelope being sent off to a faraway lab, where pathologists somehow more expert than the ones at Penn would hover over this perplexing phenomenon.

Jonathan said, "Courage, man. You can do this."

I nodded. We tried to smile. We gave each other the soul-brother shake.

"Every day in every way I'm getting better and better." The mantra returned to me, despite the circumstances, or because of them.

In the silence we braced ourselves for the worst, hoping for the best, paralyzed in the space between them.

Jonathan choked out, "You already survived the hardest part."

He was right. In my mind, the cancer was already becoming a secondary issue, this diagnosis a distraction from the primary matter at hand—my cracked chest and precious pig-intestine graft. I still had some serious healing to do.

Just after Dr. Dan Landsburg left, my friend Dr. Dan Peterson entered. The two docs, one in lab coat, the other in flannel shirt and corduroys, must have crossed paths in the hallway. I imagined them exchanging wary glances, Dan Peterson reading the exiting doctor's somber expression.

I told him—*lymphoma*. He didn't show surprise, though he must have been remembering the countless late-night hours he'd spent at the computer, investigating my symptoms and meticulously refuting the various working diagnoses. There was no argument now. We all sat quietly. The final report loomed in a future that seemed to grow darker. Dan reminded me that there were many kinds of lymphoma—a fact that deepened my sense of dread, though he meant to be encouraging.

I called my dad, who took the news stoically. He would start with phone calls to his oncologist friends, he told me. It was not long before he called back. His oncologist friends predicted "diffuse large B-cell lymphoma," which presents in the mediastinum, as mine had, and is very treatable, even curable.

Dr. Trerotola had gotten wind of the diagnosis and popped in to say hello. "So, lymphoma, huh?" he said.

I was puzzled by his apparent enthusiasm. "Why are you so pleased?" I asked. "Everyone thought it was benign."

For a moment he seemed puzzled himself by my failure to grasp the obvious. He said, "Well, it's *treatable*."

I felt faintly encouraged, understanding that for this man of science the situation had evolved into territory that finally made sense; once a problem was identified, a plan to seek a solution could be made.

· · ·

On Friday Dr. Dan Landsburg returned. He sat before my parents, Vana, and me. Again, he didn't waste time. He said, "So, you have diffuse large B-cell lymphoma."

For a moment there was a dreadful silence, until my dad gave me the thumbs-up, his eyes already watery with gratitude and relief.

The words echoed in my mind; *diffuse large B-cell . . . curable.*

Dan explained the course of chemotherapy for this kind of non-Hodgkin's lymphoma. As soon as we could get started, chemo would be administered. As an outpatient, I'd be in and out in a matter of hours, once every three weeks, six times over the course of the next four months. He described the so-called port to be implanted directly into the chest, right into the SVC, so that the chemicals could instantly enter the heart and be disseminated rapidly throughout the body.

We had questions. What about the graft healing inside of me? Could it endure the cell-destroying power of chemo? And must the chemo be channeled directly through a port inserted right into my SVC, which wasn't even really my SVC anymore, but a fragile tube crafted out of pig intestine? I pictured clouds of poison entering my chest, like napalm, hot-pink and indifferent.

I asked, "Shouldn't we wait until my graft heals completely?"

"You don't wait three months to treat someone with cancer," Dan said. "The good news is that yours is an aggressive lymphoma, which responds well to chemo even if it is late-stage."

Aggressive cancer didn't sound like good news to me.

"I'm recommending a young oncologist," Dan said. "He's your age, a really cool guy I think you'll hit it off with. I can get you in to see him on short notice, possibly even before you leave the hospital."

I asked, "Who's the best, not the coolest?"

Dan grinned. "Schuster. But he's much busier."

My dad promptly jotted down the name. "That's who we want. Schuster."

Dan nodded. "I'll get back to you with answers to your other questions. In the meantime, go home. Rest. Be with your family."

I stood, and we shook hands. As appealing as home sounded, the prospect of leaving the hospital again without answers was unnerving. I felt safe here.

· · ·

I was wheeled into the basement for one last CAT-scan before discharge. Vana stood beside my gurney in the otherwise empty waiting area when, suddenly, Dr. Miller, the chief of radiology, walked by.

"Dr. Miller!" I called out.

He turned, his eyes alive with recognition, though he remained silent. Perhaps word of my diagnosis, or even of my survival, had not reached him down here where the radiologists did their solitary work.

"You've heard? Lymphoma," I announced, almost gleefully, our confounding mystery at last solved.

His nod turned into an undisguised shaking of the head. He remained at a distance.

"I don't think it's lymphoma," he said.

"What?"

"I think it's a sarcoma."

Vana blurted, "That's *worse.*"

"But it was removed," he reassured us.

I sat up on my gurney. "Have you told anyone this? They're about to treat me for lymphoma."

Dr. Miller did not seem disturbed by this prospect, though to me this was a major revelation—cause for combat, I would think, between opposing clinicians, the chief radiologist duking it out with the chief pathologist.

"You *have* to treat for lymphoma," he said, oddly at ease.

"But you don't believe it's lymphoma."

"No, no—yes. If that's what the pathology report says, then—" He was searching for the right way to put this. "Had I thought it was lymphoma—" He spoke quietly, almost incoherently. "I would have advised . . . a . . . needle biopsy, avoiding invasive surgery."

"A what? But Dr. Trerotola—" Nobody would dare to touch me with a needle, I wanted to remind him. So even if we could turn back time, even knowing what we know now—

Vana pressed, "You think surgery could have been avoided?"

Dr. Miller sighed. "It's my fault if it's lymphoma. It just doesn't look like it." He was reporting to us in the present tense, as if we were back there in the lab, where the narrow tunnel of my SVC shrank to nearly nothing on the dark screen, all of us gazing at this inadequate crystal ball. "It never presents like this."

Vana and I quietly nodded. *Never. And yet—*

Dr. Miller concluded, "But you have to treat for lymphoma. If that's what the pathologists say it is, then that's what it is."

He walked off, leaving us in a mix of puzzlement and relief.

"Did that just happen?" Vana let out.

We stared at each other, our mouths agape, not quite grinning, not quite terrified by the prospect of a misdiagnosis. We began quickly to recognize what we'd just been witness to, a master practitioner coming to grips with the rare experience of having missed the call— not that he should have, or even could have, correctly made the call. After all, *it never presents like this.*

· · ·

On Friday they boosted my Coumadin dose, and by Saturday my INR—the number measuring my blood's anticoagulation level—hit the target range. All my doctors and nurses emphasized to me how crucial it was that my blood stay properly anti-coagulated so that it could travel past the surgical site without clotting. And just like that they were all wishing me well, ready for new patients on their way with fresh wounds from surgery. The IV pole, which had been by my side for weeks, was gone, Coumadin pills having replaced bags of heparin.

I was untethered. Home soon, without doctors and nurses attending to my every need. I breathed in, *Every day, in every way.* I breathed out, *I'm getting better and better.* I included another prayer from my repertoire, breathing in, *Lord Jesus Christ, Son of God,* breathing out, *have mercy on me, a sinner.* Before long, the prayers merged, *Every day in every way... have mercy on me a sinner.* I realized the syllables lined up. I counted them out on my fingertips. *Fifteen.* I felt the seconds turning into minutes. I timed my prayers. Seven rounds took ten minutes. Just like that, an hour had passed. I supposed this was meditation, pleased I'd found this mind-clearing method to see me through the hours and days ahead. The words intertwined. *Every day in Son of God have mercy on me and better... Lord Jesus Christ in every way I'm getting better a sinner...* The meanings of the words blurred; it was all the same prayer. I floated into the world beyond the hospital doors. Uncharted space.

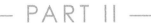

PART II

I have no desire to suffer twice, in reality and then in retrospect.

—Sophocles, *Oedipus Rex*

In our adventures, we have only seen our monster more clearly and described his scales and fangs in new ways—ways that reveal a cancer cell to be, like Grendel, a distorted version of our normal selves.

—Harold Varmus

13

TREE OF LIFE

After three days at home, my recovery was going swiftly. My chest pain was tolerable, the wound, healing. I managed showers symptom-free. I slept upright in bed, propped up by pillows. During the day I read on the couch and took short walks. I was fed extravagantly by my wife, sister, mom, and mother-in-law.

On the fourth day, when I bent over to tie my shoes, I felt a rush of blood surging into my head. I sat up. Maybe I was imagining things. I bent over to tie the other shoe. There was no mistaking it. Was I clotting up due to improper dosing of Coumadin? I didn't want to worry Vana, who was down the hallway with Nikitas in his bedroom. I tiptoed downstairs and, in a quiet voice, left a message for Dr. Pochettino, describing my unnerving symptoms and imploring him to call me back as soon as possible. Then I got back to my daytime routine of sitting in the green recliner in the living room and staring out the window.

Before noon, my mother arrived in grand style, and in a parade of trips to and from the car lugged bags of food and household products, aluminum foil and twelve-packs of paper towels from Costco. I sat tight, not bending to pick up my laptop or a book or a pillow—let alone a bag of groceries—dreading the confounding return of that pre-surgery congestion.

Vana cheered, "Oh my God, Mom, thank you!" with each delivery. Vana hadn't yet returned to work. She wanted to wait until I was through at least the first round of chemo, the date of which remained undetermined. In the meantime, her boss encouraged her not to think about the office. So, in the mornings she took Nikitas to daycare, in the afternoons she picked up groceries and cooked, and otherwise she took care of me.

I smiled from the couch, conveying to my mother with all the excitement I could muster that I could not be happier about the case of twenty-four convenient squirt bottles of spring water—not to mention the broiled salmon and potatoes she'd whipped up this morning for dinner tonight. Vana sighed in relief as my mom set the warm serving tray on the kitchen counter.

This was my mother in full form. If we didn't distract her, she would begin cleaning the house. In a few days the place would be immaculate. For decades my mom had managed to fool her children into believing that she loved doing housework in other people's homes, loved babysitting for days on end—especially if she got to drive from Lancaster to Philadelphia to do it. "You're lucky I love to drive," she beamed, and we were convinced she was telling the truth.

After the groceries were put away, my mom and I headed out for my daily walk, which meant shuffling down to the corner where the Barnes Museum was still under construction. By now I'd nearly convinced myself that the earlier return of symptoms had been a trick of the mind, the surging blood in the head no more significant than the pressure one normally feels bending over to touch his toes. Still, I clenched the phone in my pocket, making sure I didn't miss a call from Dr. Pochettino. My mother and I chitchatted about the neighborhood, admiring the progress it had made since I'd moved into the townhouse when I was a young teacher eager to turn his rent money into a mortgage, at the peak of a buyer's market. Fifteen years later, swanky condos had gone up across the street; a City Sports gym overlooked the parking lot of the Whole Foods; a Starbucks took the place of the unoccupied apartment building on the corner across from the world-class museum due to open in the spring—all within two blocks of my front door.

"You've had a lot of good years here," she said.

Before the recent turn of events, this is where the conversation would have turned toward the prospects of our moving to the suburbs, once Nikitas approached kindergarten age, or once Vana got pregnant with a second child. But today we didn't talk of future plans.

"Can we slow down?" I asked. "You're walking too fast."

She laughed, then realized I wasn't joking, which made her laugh a little more, only with a sadness in her voice. She took my arm as we passed the Whole Foods.

"I want to make it all the way today." I paused to catch my breath.

She waited for me to elaborate.

"To the corner," I said.

She studied my face to see if I was being ironic.

"Halfway there," I said. "Next week, all the way around the block."

She mirrored my grin.

When we returned home, Vana announced that the two of us needed to get out of the house to see a movie. "We can do this," she said. "It will be an adventure."

It was time to come clean. "I need to tell you—this morning I felt my head . . . when I bent over to tie my shoes."

"Oh," my mother let out, tearing up.

Vana took a deep breath. "How do you feel?"

"No symptoms." I didn't tell them I'd been exercising impeccable posture since that frightful episode hours ago. "I'm waiting for a call back from Pochettino."

"Okay." Vana's look stayed determined.

I felt compelled to fill the silence, to match her determination with some stoic expression of my own. "We can still go."

Vana grabbed her purse. Nikitas was at daycare, and my mom

would stay at the house while we were gone. We decided we had the emotional stamina to take on Terrence Malick's three-and-a-half-hour epic *The Tree of Life*. My mother wiped her tears, pleased to see us heading out on the town, happy to pretend we were a normal couple taking in a matinee.

Vana and I were two of six people in the theater, giddy as kids, with candy in a Ziploc. During the previews, the phone buzzed in my pocket. I stepped into the lobby to take a call from the hospital. It was the attending fellow on the line. He said he'd received my message describing the symptoms and he'd already discussed the matter with Dr. Pochettino.

"I'm not surprised," he said, "since the CAT-scan that was taken before your discharge shows a narrowing of the SVC."

I nearly choked on my popcorn. Still, I figured this doctor had his facts backward, recalling my symptoms from *before* surgery. I informed him of the confusion. He said, no, in the CAT-scan taken just days ago, there was absolutely a narrowing of the graft.

How was it possible that nobody had mentioned this to me before I left the hospital?

The attending fellow told me to go directly to Penn, tenth floor Silverstein building, the same wing where I'd spent last week recovering. They had a room for me.

My neck felt suddenly more swollen, my head thicker. I waved to Vana in the dark theater. Choked-up, I asked the cashier, chatting casually with the young man selling snacks, for my money back. "I have a medical issue," I said. He apologized and swiped Vana's credit card. We left, sad and quiet. All we'd wanted was to feel, just for a few hours, like people with normal lives.

I could hardly form the words to explain to Vana this strange news. Why would they have withheld this most crucial information? Why would they have sent me home?

When we entered the townhouse, my mother was wiping cabinets while cooking in the kitchen. Nikitas was sleeping in his crib upstairs. In minutes I stood at the bottom of the steps with my gym bag strapped over my shoulder, ready to depart. This was not *deja vu*. I recognized my life's unfortunate unwinding, returning me to these moments when I was kissing my little boy goodbye and hugging my mother at the door of my immaculate home.

14

GRAFTS AND STENTS AND CHEMOTHERAPY

i. Grafts

From my hospital-room bed, I wanted to cry out, "Why did you let me leave this place!"—as if somehow just staying here would have prevented this setback.

Dr. Pochettino stood in the doorway, nodding sympathetically. He explained that stenosis—this kind of narrowing—was all part of the unpredictable healing process.

Just like that, it seemed we were back where we started, give or take a cancer diagnosis, which now seemed a distant priority. If blood couldn't get to my heart, who cared about cancer?

He said that because I'd had no symptoms before being discharged, no one had told me about the narrowing of the SVC. The hope, or even assumption, was that the narrow dilation would in time widen to its intended fifteen-millimeter circumference. He said he'd be back again soon to check on me. In the meantime, he said, I was surviving just fine with a five-millimeter opening.

Five millimeters? No wider than that toothpick passageway.

They'd already gotten me on heparin, my blood properly anti-coagulated, my INR in the target zone. Trusty IV pole in hand, I headed into the hallway of Silverstein Ten, where patients fresh from surgery came to recover. Despite my relative youth, I felt like the veteran, a resident, not a visitor. I walked briskly from west to east and back again, wanting to believe that I might expand my SVC by huffing and puffing. Days passed. They told me I'd be staying here until there was a plan. They promised that this time they wouldn't let me go home until my symptoms were gone, which meant that my SVC would either open—or *be opened*.

· · ·

Dr. Trerotola was back to talk about what might come next. He described the stainless-steel stent as a thimble-size Chinese finger trap, inserted into the vessel, then expanded from the inside by an inflated balloon. He explained that the stent was a clot-magnet—a paradoxical little fix, sparing me an imminent life-threatening clot for the price of future clots. I pictured thickening blood jamming up on the jagged banks of a narrowing stream.

We sat side by side in my hospital room. On a blank piece of paper, he sketched blueprints of the procedure he anticipated. He drew theoretical pictures of my anatomy. "You've been dealt a bad hand, but you can't give up now." He pointed to the framed pictures of my wife and son nearby. "You have to do it for them."

It had never occurred to me to give up. But now I knew we were into something heavier than all that had come before. His compassionate stare sank into me. I imagined he was thinking of himself in my place, pictures of his own kids on the shelf.

He said we were going to delay intervening for ten more days, giving us close to a month of healing. The countdown was on. The date had been set. The procedure had been scheduled so that Dr. Pochettino would be available in case of an emergency. This news both scared and comforted me.

"The problem is we don't know what we're dealing with, and we won't know if you need a stent until we do the actual venogram. I'll be prepared with all my tools, everything I might need, and I'll do what I have to do, depending on what the venogram shows. Once I begin the procedure, there's no stopping."

He raised his eyebrows, to be sure I understood. He was asking me to trust him.

I nodded.

"The CAT-scan shows a compression of the SVC, presumably caused by post-surgical inflammation, which should shrink in time. That's why we're going to wait. But we can't wait too long."

Or else it could close.

He went on, "My hope is that I can place the stent all the way down, past the smaller veins, so it's only in the SVC. But—" He hesitated.

Here was the part where I needed to trust him completely.

"If the compression is occurring *above* the confluence, where the SVC meets the brachiocephalic veins, I'll have to use *two* stents, one that opens the SVC and one that opens one of the brachiocephalic veins."

"What about the other—?"

"The other brachiocephalic vein would have to be sacrificed. But remember, you'll form collaterals. The blocked blood flow will find its way through another vein—" He traced the route with his index finger, over his shoulder— "around your head, behind your brain, and back to the heart." He gave me an encouraging pat on the shoulder and after a moment slipped out the door.

• • •

Hunched over Dr. Trerotola's sketches, I looked up to discover Dr. Pochettino standing in the shadowy doorway. "The stent is a last resort," he said. "We will not do the procedure unless it is absolutely necessary. I don't want you to get a stent any more than you do."

I took a deep breath and exhaled.

He reminded me that scarring was part of the healing process.

Think of a gash on the skin, he said, how the scab hardens and shrinks, as scar tissue tightens up. No different on the inside. He reminded me how, anticipating this fibrosis, he'd crafted the graft to measure over twenty millimeters in circumference, seven wider than the existing SVC, assuming it would shrink to fifteen, forming a perfect cylinder. But now, there was no telling how much more it might narrow, or how rapidly.

"I called CorMatrix this morning," he added.

He let this news settle in; my surgeon had called the people who had created the material he'd used to make the graft, which, if it worked as anticipated, would be resorbed into my body and replaced by my own cells. Now we had questions for them. *How much time was necessary for the graft to heal? Could it endure a stent? How would it respond to chemotherapy? Did they have records of patients who had undergone such treatment?*

I didn't confess that I'd called CorMatrix that morning myself and gotten no response. Nor did I admit that my dad had also called to no avail.

"It's okay to start chemo after one month," Dr. Pochettino said. "So on Friday, after the venogram, we will start."

I was stunned. "But you said three months—"

"We *can* start it," he said, "as long as Dr. Schuster wants to."

"You said yourself Schuster wants to start chemo as soon as possible. He'd start today if it were up to him." What did I know? I hadn't even met my oncologist yet.

Dr. Pochettino nodded politely.

I repeated the clinical lessons I'd learned directly from him. "What about waiting six weeks for eighty-percent healing? Time for endothelialization to occur."

He smiled warmly at his faithful patient, his dutiful student. "The company says only three or four weeks of healing is necessary to be safe. It's enough time for full cell growth on the graft to occur."

"What if I have to get a stent? We still start the chemo?"

"Hopefully you will not need a stent."

An optimist.

"I called CorMatrix this morning," I said. "I didn't leave a message. My dad left two."

Dr. Pochettino held his smile, receiving my confession. "I promise I will talk to Dr. Schuster again. We all want the best for you."

He stepped into the fluorescent glow of the hallway. I shuffled back to my bed.

· · ·

When I awoke from an unplanned nap, Vana was sitting in a chair against the wall. My bed inclined, our eyes met on the same plane. It seemed her eyes had just opened, too.

She smiled. "Hello."

"Hi."

Her giant blue purse sat in the chair next to her.

"How long have you been here?" I asked.

"Not long. Twenty minutes."

Her folded hands rested on her lap.

"I think I fell asleep, too," she said. "I could sleep for a week."

I shifted in my bed and patted the narrow space beside me. "Let's."

She walked over, first to the left side of the bed, where she discovered my IV pole and the tube snaking heparin into my blood; then to the right, where she sat down, in the clear. "Any word from CorMatrix?"

I shook my head no. She took my hand into hers. I told her of the morning's visits. I reached for the crinkled piece of paper on the side table. I showed her the drawings by Dr. Trerotola, providing the best explanation I could.

She gazed at the sketches, a frenzy of blue ink—downward-pointing arrows between emphatically drawn walls, one stent followed by another, an expendable vein scribbled-out.

"No one wants to do a stent," I said. "Only if it's absolutely necessary. That's the good news *and* the bad news."

"How will they know if it's necessary?"

I grinned wryly. "I'll have to tell them."

She put her fingertips to the veins on my neck. "How do you feel?"

I shrugged. "The same."

"How can you stand this? The waiting."

"Beats the alternative," I said.

She blanched.

I said, "Going home too soon again, I mean."

"Yeah." She smiled sheepishly. "We don't want that."

"I won't let them discharge me until spring, if necessary," as if this were a pronouncement she should be thrilled with.

She let out a long breath. "There's this panel I'm supposed to moderate for work. Successful alumnae talking to undergraduate women. They told me don't worry about it."

"Do you *want* to do it?"

"This seems like the worst time."

"Maybe it's the best time—the perfect way to ease back into work."

"What if I lose it up there, while I'm asking questions? You're all I think about."

"Maybe that's why you should do it. Take your mind off all of this."

"I don't want to take my mind off all of this. I *can't* take my mind off all of this."

I hesitated. "I think it would be good. To think about other things. See how it feels. You're not going to lose it. You'll be great."

"I don't know." She looked around, as if trying to trace something to the source. "I can't stand the odor anymore. The antibacterial soap. The sanitizer. Whatever it is. I wash my hands as soon as I get home to get rid of the smell of this place."

I smiled.

She didn't seem to know whether to laugh or cry.

I thought, *This place is keeping me alive.* But I'd learned to keep such insufferable expressions of gratitude to myself, sensitive as I could be to her plight of feeling alone, at home, or with Nikitas, or even with the company of her mother, or mine, just waiting to see what the future would bring. Why should she or anyone else identify the hospital with anything other than pain and suffering?

"If you do the panel," I said, "it doesn't mean you have to go back to work yet, unless you decide you want to, which I think would be great."

The truth was I couldn't stomach the antiseptic stink any longer, either, and I couldn't imagine how she felt when she exited the building every day. My contentment with being here indefinitely must have deepened her sense of isolation, of her own kind of quarantine from normality, no matter where she was. Meanwhile, to me this tube tethered to my arm was more like an umbilical cord than a nuisance, and I was in no hurry to be free from it.

"I feel so disconnected," she said, "not just from work. From everything."

I shifted another inch and laid my arm out along the pillow.

"I think you should do the panel," I said.

She set the diagrams back on the side table, lifted her legs onto the bed, and rested her head next to mine, until it was time for her to go.

• • •

Beyond the white curtain, my roommate, Vinnie, unhitched from his IV pole, couldn't wait to get out of here. His discharge papers were being processed, he said, though he was pacing as if he didn't really trust the plan. The night before, his wife brought dinner from their Italian restaurant in New Jersey. We ate gnocchi, chicken, and salad, as Vinnie told me his story. He'd been in a coma for eleven days, and now he suffered from withdrawal. He'd agreed to treatment for drug addiction. He didn't think the heparin drip was sufficient cause for his continued stay, and evidently, they acquiesced. I warned him not to leave prematurely, as if he hadn't already made up his mind.

In the bathroom I examined my neck veins. The shadows made them appear bloated and bluish. With a fingertip I traced their bulging path from clavicle to jawbone. I dreaded the seeming inevitability of a stent and of the complications that would follow. I stretched my neck to see the lines flatten, and I felt some relief. In a dimmer light the veins appeared normal, and hours passed without a flicker of discomfort.

Not long after Vinnie was gone, my new roommate entered—a talker. My merciful nurse whispered to me that she'd reserved the single that had just been vacated at the far end of the hall. Later, on my walk to my new digs, IV pole in tow, I could see that the window on the far wall framed the city skyline. The room was a veritable suite. The nurse must have had a hunch that I would be spending at least the next month here.

ii. Stents

The nurse practitioner said, "If it closes up, you could code," as in *code blue*, doctor slang for cardiac arrest, "and then we've got a serious emergency on our hands, and we don't want that."

"I'm getting used to this feeling of being gently strangled." I meant to sound reassuring, not dramatic.

Her ice-blue eyes bored into me. "Don't get *too* used to it."

"I mean, I'm willing to live in the hospital indefinitely," I said, "until spring if you let me—however long it takes. March, April. I don't care." I wanted everyone to understand. Do not do me any favors and rush to send me home again.

"Let's hope you're not still here in April," she said.

"Let's hope."

I wore jeans and a hoodie to feel at home, which was what this place had become for me. At times I felt strangely blissful, my life having been distilled to its essence, despite my separation from the physical reality of it—or because of it. When I walked up and down the hallway, I was aware of each breath, smiling and nodding hello to the nurses and doctors. When I ate, I was mindful of each bite. Some nights Jonathan Rubin brought food from a neighborhood restaurant—sushi, Thai, pizza. We watched baseball. Every afternoon I met Vana and Nikitas in the lobby, where Nikitas was learning to walk. I took his hand in my free one, IV pole in the other, as we scurried on the linoleum floor. Vana took videos I would watch later on my iPhone. When Lee and Alex visited from New York, I took them on a tour, to the cafeteria, to the courtyard. Back in my room, I spoke with doctors in a language my friends couldn't comprehend, talking INRs and SVCs, grafts and stents and chemotherapy; they looked at me as though I'd been living in another country, having returned bilingual.

· · ·

I was sitting at my window when an unfamiliar doctor in a white coat arrived. I twisted to see his eyes smiling over brown horn-rimmed glasses, his peppery mat of hair wispy over his ears. "Dr. Schuster," I realized. We shook hands. Until now I knew him only as the oncologist I should hope to get. He said he wanted to hear my whole story. He listened patiently. When he said that Dr. Pochettino wanted to delay treatment to let the graft heal, I understood he was inviting my thoughts. I appreciated that I was not only my own advocate but also the crucial mediator, triangulating these voices and influencing outcomes. He said he was willing to stretch out the healing for as long as possible. "We're not waiting any more than six weeks," he said. "Eight weeks or three months? Forget it. You'll be coming back here with other problems."

"I understand."

"I looked at the latest CAT-scan. I'm not convinced a stent will be necessary."

I felt a rush of relief.

He added, "I'm not convinced the narrowing of the SVC is being caused by post-surgical inflammation," as the theory went.

"Then what?"

"By lymphoma," he said—by a tumor that had already developed since the surgery.

I was stunned by the prospect of cancer growing inside me again, as if it had ever been completely vanquished.

"Yours is an aggressive cancer," he reminded me, "but this also means it will respond well to treatment."

I nodded, though I was unnerved, not only by this theory of a growing tumor but by the apparent conflict between my doctors, their opinions at odds. And then I reminded myself how, for better or worse, the man with the hammer sees a nail, which he can pound with his distinctive tool; the surgeon sees what he can repair with his scalpel; the oncologist, what he can treat with his medicine—a clear solution, if only in theory. In my case, it was a theory that meant avoiding a stent. So just like that, I was strangely hopeful that the cause of my constricted blood flow was the return of a tumor—a tumor that, this time, would be eliminated with chemotherapy.

· · ·

The next day I was being wheeled off to the oncology wing of the Rhoads Building, a long, winding ride that led to a quiet, peaceful hallway. Each room was a single. Patients rested behind closed doors and pulled curtains. Doctors and nurses did their work at the long main desk, hunched at computers or studying clipboards. Vana and my parents, brother, and sister hauled my collected belongings and assembled them on the windowsill, which overlooked a stony walkway lined with oak trees. Across the way stood the medical school. Beyond the windows, students worked together at tables and alone in cubicles. I settled in comfortably.

Instead of going for a stent—or for the scheduled venogram,

which was now deemed unnecessary—I started on prednisone, prelude to chemotherapy, two giant horse pills they promised would make me full of energy I wouldn't know how to use, and possibly mood swings I wouldn't know how to combat. The hope was that the drug would have an anti-inflammatory effect and that we would begin to see the veins in my neck less distended. By early afternoon doctors were peeking in to check on progress. One of the oncology fellows said he didn't want to get our hopes up, but he thought my veins looked smaller. *Obviously wishful thinking*, an opinion I kept to myself every time I returned to the mirror in the bathroom. I didn't want to be seen as the pessimistic patient who needed a pep talk.

After four doses of prednisone, my symptoms remained the same. So now it was up to the chemotherapy, which I'd be starting tomorrow—four hours of IV drips and "pushes"—medicines pushed into the veins through a large vial.

Earlier in the day an ultrasound of my armpit had been done, after I complained of a pain that came from a taut tendon, tender to the touch. The theory, upon investigation, was that there was clotting of small superficial veins. But at the moment no one seemed especially interested in this inconsequential matter, myself included. We had bigger fish to fry.

iii. Chemotherapy

Another week had passed since my arrival in Rhoads room 3005. I lay in bed watching the IV slowly doing its work. Mom, Dad, and Vana sat quietly in the corners, mostly reading. They picked at a pizza they'd brought from some nearby joint. They glanced up, smiling politely, as if anticipating shrieks of pain, though they saw that I was practically enjoying myself here, or I was pretending to be, hamming it up every time a doctor poked his head in and offered a chummy nod and a "How's it going?" The truth was that, perhaps like my audience, I was disguising a fear that the poison coursing through my body might begin to destroy the graft in my chest. I gave them all a big thumbs-up and said, "Keeping it together!" or "Still intact!"

My dad offered me a slice of pizza, but I'd been warned of nausea and wasn't in the mood for food. Somehow, though, I was in the mood for music, so I listened to Springsteen's *Darkness on the Edge of Town* on my headphones. I texted my friend Matt in Nashville to tell him I had his favorite Bruce album going during my first treatment. He aptly replied, "Is there any life experience not improved with a Bruce playlist?" I dozed off before the last drops had made their way through the IV attached to my arm. When I awoke, I was surprised to feel normal—and hungry. I ate pizza from the box, as well as most of my dinner from the cafeteria.

At night I managed to watch baseball, happy to see Albert Pujols and the Cardinals enjoying their push toward the NL championship. The Phils didn't deserve it, I realized, in awe of the four remaining teams, whose young and quick players hammered the ball. Our Phils and those Yanks now seemed like tired old guys, injured and trying to mend. It was a year for youthful vitality.

The next morning—October 16th, exactly two months since that first flare-up—the chemo began to match its reputation. Nausea set in. I couldn't eat. I couldn't read. I contemplated the stack of untouched tomes I'd brought from home—*The Joseph Campbell Companion*, Whitman's *Leaves of Grass*—whose presence alone, on my makeshift nightstand, had been providing me the comfort I'd planned to get from reading them.

At lunchtime I couldn't bear the sight or smell of what had arrived on the cafeteria tray. I managed to eat some of the soup Vana brought, one of her mom's concoctions, a translucent orangey broth that relieved me of my nausea.

When Dr. Schuster gave me the green light to go home, he was surprised that I didn't want to leave. I reminded him that I'd been at a similar crossroads before and that I wanted to be in the clear this time. "You're in command," he said.

Alone, I felt suddenly depressed, thinking about my symptoms, which were the same I'd had two months ago—neck veins puffed-up and head congested. I sat in the recliner by the window, breathing quietly, trying to lose myself in the trees and sky. *Every day in every way I'm getting better and better.*

When Vana called to say she and Nikitas were on their way, I donned the flannel hoodie my sister had brought me from J. Crew. She had supplied me with a hospital wardrobe to rival the one that filled my closet at home. With each visit, she pulled new items from giant bags—T-shirts, button-downs, long-sleeve jerseys, pajama bottoms, boxer shorts—displaying them for my approval before tossing them onto the bed. I was the Jay Gatsby of the oncology wing.

Geared up for fall weather, I walked outside in the idyllic tree-lined area between the hospital and medical school. This had become the daily routine. After work, Vana would pick up Nikitas at daycare and then "go to the park" to see Daddy. I rushed toward them, IV pole in hand, the whole wheeled contraption skipping and skidding beside me on the path. To us city dwellers, this area was like a nature preserve. Nikitas sat in the dirt playing with sticks. "Squail," he said, at the flash of a gray furry question mark in the grass. *Squirrel.* He was not only walking and talking now, but he was thoughtful and playful and creative, his gears turning at every moment, his curiosity and compassion triggered by the simplest cues. An hour in the dirt with my boy and all had improved, so much so that I considered going home, despite whatever risks, lamenting the hours and minutes I was not with him. He fingered the thin tube snaking under the tape on my arm. He kissed my boo-boo and pointed out more moving creatures.

• • •

I was eating dinner, or poking at a pale piece of chicken, when my mom surprised me with a visit. She said she was in town helping Vana for a few days. I didn't know who was where from one day to the next anymore. I set my fork down. My mother smiled. She seemed to be gauging my mood, pondering the effects of the chemicals in my bloodstream. Perhaps she understood, long before I did, that I needed to get the hell out of there.

At dusk we went for a walk outside in the enclosed courtyard. When we returned to the building, the glass doors were locked. The well-lit hallway was empty for a minute, until a large group, apparently generations of the same family, led by a bald and goateed father in a rugby shirt, began streaming past. My mother and I knocked, as one after another passed—several young couples, their children, an old man. They saw us. I knocked a little harder. They pointed at the warning signs and stickers, explaining over their shoulders that they were forbidden to open the doors, that the alarms would ring.

My mother chuckled, curious about what would come next. She had no idea. Neither did I, but I felt myself being transported by swelling waves of emotion.

"What the hell," I muttered.

"It's okay," my mother assured me.

My agitation boiled. *Do these people think I'm trying to break into this place? With my fucking IV pole and my septuagenarian mother? Are they not getting the visual clues that I belong on the inside, not the outside, of this building? Can they not infer that I'm the expert here, I'm the veteran, I've been here six fucking weeks, and I know that alarms do not sound even when the doors are opened after-hours? Don't they know I'm the one with cancer who almost bit the dust, and still might, and* "Open the fucking door already!"

It was only when the old man opened the door and said, "There's no need for that kind of language," that I understood how my outrage had erupted, just as the young father in the rugby shirt asked his wife what kind of a human being could speak in such a way, with children around. It was a good thing, his wife said to me, that I was already in the hospital. Up ahead toddlers in sweatsuits peered over their shoulders, their mothers or aunts or grandmothers rushing them toward the elevators, away from the pale ghoul gripping the IV pole like a spear.

Back in my room, we speculated on the woman's intended meaning, "*It's a good thing you is already in the hospital.*" My mom guessed she meant that, if I weren't already in the hospital, then her husband would have *put* me there. I believed she meant that God had already punished me, so there was no use in punishing me further.

Crying, I asked my mom when I had become this terrible person who lashed out at others like that—or was this who I really was, who I'd always been? My mother reassured me it was the prednisone. I thanked her for her generous diagnosis.

That night I downloaded *The Tree of Life* onto my new iPad. Seconds into the elaborate prologue, I decided that this was a movie that must be watched on a screen bigger than the one I could prop up on my hospital tray, and it must be watched by Vana and me together, as we'd originally intended. But then I couldn't stop watching, mesmerized by the convincing depiction of the Big Bang, then the origins of life, a boiling soupy concoction generating all on its own, in the dark depths beneath the planet's firm surface, the first living cell, then cells, conjoining and replicating inexplicably—a fish grows legs, climbs toward the light, and becomes a small dinosaur, whose life is later spared for no apparent reason by a large dinosaur. With torrents of hopeful tears streaming down my face—another side effect of the prednisone—I interpreted this act as the dawn of mercy.

· · ·

The next morning, my mom returned with Vana, who announced it was time for me to come home. I acquiesced but refused to leave before one last debriefing with Dr. Pochettino, whom I hadn't seen in days. Meanwhile, my dad understood my parting wish, which was why he'd gone straight to Silverstein Ten, where on Thursdays, my surgeon made his rounds. Moments later my father entered the room, out of breath and beaming, Dr. Pochettino in tow.

Dr. Pochettino stood before us with his usual graceful confidence, even when interrupted by his cell phone, whose ring tone was the opening of Bob Seger's "Old Time Rock and Roll." His blue eyes and smile still had the power to reassure us, even as he announced that in the latest CAT-scan the graft had narrowed severely, precisely where he'd hoped it wouldn't, precisely where it should be at its widest. Instead of fifteen millimeters, it was now *less* than five.

My heart sank.

He explained that the cause of the narrowing was not a tumor after all, as the oncologists had cheerfully predicted, but simply the imperfect healing of the graft—something chemo could not fix.

He fielded a smattering of obvious, unanswerable questions: Was it safe to go home? Would the graft continue to narrow? Was I in danger? When should I go to the emergency room?

"The hope is that collateral veins will form," he said, and I could hardly believe my ears at the sound of the once-promising words given by Dr. Woo upon my discharge back in August.

Now I needed something more than hope, but I wasn't sure what it was.

Other familiar questions followed. How long would it take for collaterals to form? Would they form before the graft closed up or I needed a stent?

Dr. Pochettino offered what little reassurance he could, before rising from the wall he'd been leaning against. He asked if we had any more questions, then left the room.

I finally understood what I needed—something a surgeon couldn't provide.

• • •

Dr. Weinrieb had paid me a brief visit back in Silverstein Ten—a friendly pop-in arranged by Peter Bloom, my dad's retired psychiatrist friend. Pretty savvy, that Peter Bloom, who had given me Dr. Weinrieb's phone number, playing up how he thought I would like him—you know, just a good guy who happened to be a psychiatrist, if you ever feel like talking to someone, as things develop down the road.

Now, days after chemo, I felt myself unraveling, needing to talk to someone other than a family member or a friend. I was feeling alone, despite the company, about to confront my ambiguous prognosis beyond the safe walls of the hospital.

Dr. Weinrieb responded promptly to my call, arriving after everyone cleared out of my room. He closed the door and took the seat in the corner. He smiled and rested his hands on his knees. "So," he said—and that's all I needed. I ranted about the irony of my current situation, how I'd returned to where I'd started, once again hoping for collaterals. Now part pig intestine, my SVC had narrowed exactly where my old SVC had been blocked by a mysterious mass that turned out to be lymphoma, which we were now treating with chemo, and which had nothing to do with the symptoms I once again had.

We talked about control, and my lack of it. He talked about how my strength had now become my weakness—how I'd played a prominent role in my own health care, learning a whole new vocabulary, reading CAT-scans, and comparing images, influencing doctors in their treatment, nudging, and clarifying and guiding their care for me toward my recovery. But now there was nothing I could do but to let go, to let my body heal on its own, to wait for my vascular system to perform its greatest miracle—to form new and expanded pathways from pre-existing veins—and to trust that this miracle might happen before my new vein, the most important vein in the body, narrowed to a point that would require intervention, or sealed up without notice.

"Okay, let's slow down for a moment," Dr. Weinrieb said.

I listened and did as he instructed.

"Breathe deep. Imagine a place that gives you comfort."

The beach.

"Think of every detail. Really feel those details."

The sand. The waves. The clouds. The dunes.

"Imagine one of those thermometers from way back—the kind they used to have in classrooms when you were little. Now imagine that red ball going down, down, down, from 100, to 90. Now count down from 10, 9, 8 . . . See and feel how you're okay. You're still okay. The symptoms are real, yes, maybe even worse. But you're still okay. And then tomorrow it's the same, or maybe even a little worse. But you're still here, still okay. And then you start to see your life, and your progress, in a bigger picture, seeing how the patterns allow for dips that linger, sensations that come and often go, and there's time, time for collaterals to form, or just to call for help if necessary, or to get to the hospital if necessary, but for now, right now, you're okay, and you've got my number if you need anything at all, don't hesitate, anytime, even if you just need to talk, if you just want to let off steam. Still okay."

Okay.

15

THE RISE OF CANCER BOY

The leaves had fallen from the magnolia tree outside the living room window where I'd been sitting for the past week, fantasizing about rising and journeying into the world. I monitored my worsening symptoms, my neck veins engorged, my head puffed up. The second week after chemo was the roughest, as promised. I'd no sooner gotten past the nausea than my white blood cell count dropped. For days I'd felt simultaneously heavy and light, feet weighed down and head in the stars.

Now the white cell count had started to rise. For one week I would be climbing toward normal while bracing myself for the next treatment.

My brother-in-law, Niko, called to ask if I wanted to go to the Eagles-Cowboys game. I wanted to say yes, for a moment unable to think of a reason why I shouldn't attend a football game. It would be just days after the second treatment, and I was thinking maybe the crippling nausea wouldn't have set in yet. Then I thought about the commotion in South Philly, the fans herded like cattle down the concrete ramp after the game, the shouldering and bumping, my risk of internal bleeding, lest I be too tired to cheer satisfactorily for the hometown team and be mistaken for a Cowboys fan. I told Niko maybe next season.

My first venture into the world was to attend a literary event at Bryn Mawr College, where my friend Robin was on a panel with four other writers discussing The Short Story. Robin's husband, Richard, drove all the way from the suburbs to pick me up. When I opened the door to the minivan, he smiled and said, "Hey, Cancer Boy." I was stunned, then weirdly thrilled, this nickname suggesting youth and, better yet, survival. I grinned, trusting Richard's intuition. *Cancer Boy.* It was the twisted name of a superhero, or the superhero's sidekick. I was weak-boned, pale-skinned and puffed-up, cocooned in black alpaca-hair coat and ski cap, snug atop my thinning hair. As we drove from the bright city into the dark suburban landscape, I wondered at my new identity. This was the beginning of a metamorphosis. I watched from the shadows, biding my time, grateful to be the passenger.

In the back of an old cathedral, we sat under stained-glass windows and colossal beams. Robin and the three other writers were on stage behind a long table in the far distance, beyond rows of heads. I was there, and somehow also not there, floating at the edges of a community of writers I had over the years come to belong to. Tonight, I was privately rooting for all of them, the thrill I felt for the magnificent power of words and stories undiluted by my own ambitions. Their faces glowed under spotlights—Karen Russell, Chris Adrian, Rivka Galchen—whose stories I had read with awe, these three alongside my friend Robin Black, whose modest brilliance shone brightest in my eyes. I was pleased to relinquish the creative responsibilities to them entirely. They would do what work needed to be done. It was a relief to be off the hook, to be a witness to the relevant and vital activities of the living. I did not yet recognize that my own work had become an unconscious process of collecting scraps I might one day use in the story I would have to tell.

After the presentation, while the authors signed books and others mingled, I stood against a wall, feeling ghostly despite my dark coat and olive-green cap. Dan Torday, the program director, glanced my way and didn't seem to recognize me. Then he smiled warmly and approached. He said he'd been getting reports from Robin. He invited me to join him and the visiting authors at the local pub. I had never turned down his past invitations, and tonight more than ever I wanted to drink a beer and chat idly about books, or just to inhabit the same space for a while longer, with these writers whose intelligence and creativity seemed to project outward from them, materializing in blue-green tattoos on the arms of Chris Adrian, oozing in dark tendrils from the head of Rivka Galchen, who right now, behind a nearby table stacked with paperbacks, was telling a curious woman what it was like to be both a doctor and an author.

Later, walking across the quad toward the parking lot, I told Chris that for years I'd been teaching his story, "Every Night for a Thousand Years," which features Walt Whitman, our great poet, the selfless lover, nursing soldiers back to health during the Civil War. Chris reminded me that he was also a pediatric oncologist, and I thought, who are these magnificent beings in my midst, master practitioners of medicine and fiction? I was a master practitioner of a different sort, I wanted to tell them, with insights to share from the other side.

But my energy was dwindling, and Richard's minivan was waiting. I was strangely at ease watching them all disappear into the night, pleased that our lives had intersected for this brief moment. Mine was, I realized, the thinking of an old man, pleased with the time he'd had here, content with the prospects of finality. These were not morbid thoughts, but those of sweet sorrow. While I no longer expected to die soon, I'd been left feeling the chill of the imminence of death—for all of us. My God. *Go, all of you, brilliant souls, and make beautiful things!* It is only that I may beat you to it, is all.

• • •

At my pre-treatment appointment for round two of chemo, Dr. Schuster examined the puffed-up flesh around my neck. I was increasingly symptomatic, trying to rise above the discomfort, to accept that I had bad days and less-bad days, that the swelling came and went. I was trying to reconcile this illogical, quasi-hopeful notion with the disturbing fact that the graft, in its continued healing, was shrinking and not likely to reverse course.

Vana sat anxiously in a chair against the wall of the exam room. She'd brought a photocopy of a list of healthy foods—flax seeds, et cetera. She'd been reading a book on diet designed to avoid cancer. I'd told her I already had cancer.

"It's no better," Dr. Schuster said, pressing his fingertips into my edematous flesh.

"It's worse," I said.

His entourage, comprising five young women in white lab coats like his, formed a semi-circle behind him. One sat at the computer taking notes. One held a clipboard. Dr. Schuster told the one at the computer to get Dr. Pochettino on the phone. She managed to find the number for his mobile. Dr. Schuster called from his own mobile.

"Alberto! Steve Schuster! I've got Jim Zervanos here. He's no better. Do you want to do the stent now or do you want to wait until I finish the full treatment of chemo in six months?"

Do the stent? I was stunned. I anticipated Dr. Pochettino's hopeful reply. When Dr. Schuster gave me the thumbs-up, I grinned, relieved. *No stent.*

Then Dr. Schuster called Dr. Trerotola. "Scott, Steve Schuster . . . If you think you're going to do a stent, I'd rather you do it now. Once I get the chemo going, I don't want to interrupt it." My eyes were locked on Dr. Schuster's. Finally, he nodded, as Dr. Trerotola confirmed that we should proceed with the chemo and hope for collaterals.

Dr. Schuster slipped his phone into his coat pocket. "All your doctors are on the same page."

I asked if he'd seen patients like me with obstructions causing collaterals to form.

He beamed. "All the time!"

"So you think that's going to happen with me?"

He pressed his horn-rimmed glasses to his face. "Absolutely! It's inevitable! It's how the venous system works. You'll see the blue veins right on your chest wall."

I asked how long it takes for these collateral veins to form.

"Six months."

I pictured blood dripping through an hourglass.

Dr. Schuster pressed his fingertips on my chest and stretched the skin, inspecting in vain for signs of collaterals already rising to the surface. He gave me an encouraging pat on the shoulder.

"Okay," Vana let out. She waited for Dr. Schuster's attention. "Should Jimmy be increasing his vitamin B17 intake?"

"I have no idea what vitamin B17 is," Dr. Schuster said. He scanned the paper Vana handed him. He promptly handed it back to her. "Avoid flax seeds, and every other food on the list, for that matter."

Vana appeared discouraged but not defeated.

Yesterday I'd received a care package from California. John Bon and his girlfriend had stuffed the box with bagged goji berries, jarred homemade concoctions, and informational pamphlets that joined the small pile of books on macrobiotics that my health-conscious friend had already sent from Amazon. We were assembling a small library that I couldn't help seeing as an ironic display of Too Little Too Late.

Vana asked, "Is it okay for him to eat things like hamburgers and chicken wings?"

Dr. Schuster looked at her, puzzled.

She went on, "We were thinking of going to our neighborhood tavern tonight. We just need to get out of the house. It's just that—"

When he looked at me suspiciously, I shrugged and shrank back, redirecting his attention to Vana, who asked, "Is it true that, since cancer needs an acidic environment to grow in, one could prevent it by creating an acid-free environment?"

Dr. Schuster grinned and shook his head, as if to suggest he wouldn't hold this lapse in rational thought against either of us.

Danielle, his nurse practitioner, chimed in, "Many of these foods aid in *protecting* cells, and the point of chemo is to *destroy* cells, so we don't want to create an internal battle."

"Hm." Vana was reluctant to give in.

Dr. Schuster insisted, "Tonight I want you to go to the tavern for a beer and a burger."

Vana let out a long skeptical breath.

"Doctor's orders," he said, and returned my smile.

16

HAPPY BIRTHDAY

After the second chemo treatment, my hair began to thin, at first in the shower, my palms glazed with sudsy strands after I shampooed. Within days, washing my hair became an exercise in removing it, my fingers enmeshed with clumps of my locks. I was morbidly thrilled by the sensation of my body severing ties with a part of itself, as I uprooted with my own hands hair I'd never sheared to so much as a crewcut. I called out to Vana to come see. When I showed her vines of black hair falling from my fingers, she turned her head. I tried to joke, to soothe her from the sight, pretending to be insane, or to be *going* insane, making a wild face while literally pulling my hair out.

"Aren't you upset?" she asked.

I shook my head, smiling.

"I don't want you to be bald."

"Okay." I stopped pulling at it.

I didn't want to clog the drain, so I cleared my hands over the toilet. In the mirror I was shocked to see that my Greek genes had proved resilient; no one would know the difference, despite what I'd just plucked. A virtual wig, or at least toupee, sat atop the surface of the toilet water. The next day I didn't need the shampoo to lubricate the removal, which I was eager to expedite, if only to avoid the imminent patchwork look.

Out on the patio, under sunny skies, I started with the madman routine before taking it easy, working my fingers through what remained until all that was left was a shadowy remnant of my do. As an early birthday present, I had received from my father-in-law a snazzy electric razor, which I'd been instructed by my doctors to use on my face, in lieu of a blade, lest I lose control and drain myself of my anti-coagulated blood. I took my new Braun to the thatched remains of my scalp, leaving my sideburns. At my next appointment, Dr. Schuster told me to lose the chops.

For the next month I enjoyed encouraging comments. "You look amazing." "Like Vin Diesel." "As good as you do with hair." I mugged for the camera, donned black shades, and offered my baddest-ass scowl. Our Christmas card featured the three of us at the *LOVE* sculpture, all smiles. I looked like a guy who shaved his head or lost a bet. But when the eyebrows vanished and the prednisone took full effect, the compliments stopped. I looked like a guy who had cancer—pale, puffy, and hairless. I felt translucent. The looks I got in public reminded me that I had not vanished yet.

As my forty-second birthday approached, I was in surprisingly good spirits despite the aches, nausea, and baldness. Vana had planned a celebration, and I was ready to head into the city without fear of bleeding or clotting.

She started me with the royal treatment—pedicure, manicure, and facial—all firsts for me. Pampering was the idea, she said, explaining that the facial was more of a massage than a cleansing treatment. Kelly, the masseuse, tilted my head and worked her fingertips into my shoulders, neck, and scalp.

Vana had told Kelly that I'd been through two chemo treatments—and through a lot more before that. The intentional touch of a professional who was not administering chemotherapy or examining me for symptoms was a revelation. Kelly told me that she and her daughter lived in Jersey with her mother—she'd lived in South Philly until a recent bad breakup. As she spoke, her hands were a swarm of butterflies. I imagined her sorrow pouring out of her in waves of tenderness. I began to believe this "facial" might heal me. An hour later, in the hallway, she reached to shake my hand. I hugged her instead and said thank you. "You're going to be okay," she said. "I'm not even bullshitting you. I just know." I let myself believe she had a mystic's insight, as penetrating as her touch.

Vana and I had lunch at Parc, looking out over Rittenhouse Square. The nausea at bay, I felt like a normal person, even as strange waves of aches and pains flitted and lingered all over my body. Headaches came and went. Muscles knotted and relaxed. I was told that these sensations might be magnified because I was in withdrawal from oxycodone, a fact that might also explain my recent bouts of irritability and impatience, though I wasn't inclined to make excuses, especially on my birthday, when I was being treated like a prince.

• • •

Days later, I woke up feeling swollen, symptomatic. It was the day before my PET scan, which would determine whether I was on the right course of chemo. I'd been feeling well enough to be up and around—until today. Home alone, I stayed immobile in my new green chair, watching my new TV—two extraordinary birthday gifts meant to replicate the luxury I'd become accustomed to in my hospital oncology suite, where I'd sat by the window in a leather recliner with a flatscreen on the wall above the far sink. I felt congestion in my neck and head, puffed up in the area above my clavicle and even— this was new—in the small area under my chin. My flesh felt tender and taut, filled to the gills. I sucked on ginger candies, a custom carried over from the days with nausea. I wore one of five beanies I rotated for color variety. Exposed to the air, the head got cold.

When Vana got home from work, she felt tapped out. The rain

wasn't helping her mood. The storm door thumped behind her. "God *damn it*," she hissed, glistening with controlled frustration. She hauled in six bags of groceries and as many gallon jugs of spring water, setting them on the floor inside the front door. "Oh, hi," she said, when she saw me sitting in the dark, on the green chair, as if I were ever anywhere else. "I'll get all this when I get back." She headed out to park the car and then to pick up Nikitas at Bright Horizons on the corner. I tested the weight of the bags and left them there. I carried one jug to the pantry, and that was all. I returned to my chair.

When Vana returned with Nikitas in his stroller, she said he'd been calling out my name the entire way home. "Dah-dee!" he cheered. I undid his belt buckle. I wanted to play with him, but I knew my limitations. I sank back into my chair. Vana shed her damp coat and let off steam as she wiped rain mixed with perspiration from her forehead and hauled grocery bags into the kitchen while recapping the highs and lows of her day. I told her I wanted to help but couldn't. She knew today had not been good for me. She teared up. She said she'd had a bad day, too; she couldn't have a good day if she knew I was having a bad day, knowing I was sitting idle in this chair. I said it wouldn't be forever. I said I didn't mind. I wrote. I read. It was really okay. She said she was tired—*of doing everything.* I got to my feet and reached for a bag, which she grabbed first.

"Don't." She looked up, at Nikitas running toward his toys, the bags of groceries on the kitchen floor, the sink full of dishes.

"I'm sorry." I returned to my chair.

She said, "No, don't say you're sorry."

She gathered herself and went to it, starting with Nikitas's dinner. Nikitas stood between my legs at the coffee table, snacked on crackers and juice, fed me bits and pieces, as I fed him. He leaned into my legs. I palmed his belly. I played his favorite animal video on TV. He did a little dance. We said the names of the animals. We sang along with the music. His dinner was ready. Vana set up the highchair. I sat in the chair across from him, as he fingered his spinach and breaded fish. He ate some pieces. He tossed a chunk of fish onto the floor. I knew better than to bend over to pick it up, but I didn't want to be entirely useless. I stared at the fish. It seemed a mile away. I tried feeding him with my fingers. He ate a few more pieces. He was squirming, calling for something. Vana twisted at the sink, asked what he wanted. He whined, picked at his food on the tray. I glanced again at the fish on the floor. I went to pick it up.

All of a sudden my arm was undulating in the air—I could see it and feel it, understanding that it was moving all on its own, and that my head was growing light, my vision dark, and all the while I heard Vana saying, "Oh my God, what's the matter?" My arm seemed to be dancing in front of me as my head was floating off. And then, just like that, I was back, my arm still, my vision clearing.

Vana was already on the phone, saying, "I'm calling the police."

"The police?"

She cried out, "What's the number?!"

"911?"

"Yes!"

"I'm okay," I said.

"No, you're not. I'm calling your dad."

"There's nothing he can do. Believe me. I'm not going to the hospital right now."

She looked at me.

"I should have just stayed in my chair, where I felt fine all day. That was my mistake." I shuffled back to my chair, berating myself. I shouldn't have pushed myself. I'd wanted to help. I wanted to be involved.

She said, "You have to call your dad."

"Fine."

I called him. I explained to him what had just happened. I said I thought I was about to faint.

Vana took the phone. "It was more like a seizure."

My father explained that my worsened symptoms might relate to the drop in barometric pressure. News to me. He said patients who were healing often experienced swelling or shrinking of tissue during inclement weather. Going to the hospital didn't seem necessary.

Vana was skeptical but remained silent. We thanked my dad and hung up.

Vana fed Nikitas at the kitchen table. I watched them from across the room.

I checked my iPhone for the forecast. Fair tomorrow. Rain in the morning. Clear skies in the afternoon.

The phone rang. My brother, John, said he'd confirmed the reservation for tomorrow night—Butcher & Singer for our annual birthday dinner.

Vana glared at me.

I assured her, "I won't go unless I feel up to it."

I told John about the near-fainting episode. I said I'd been fantasizing about an overlarge slab of dry-aged rib eye.

Vana rolled her eyes and smirked. I blew her a kiss.

John said he'd had a bad day, too. And then, "I predict that after you get your PET-scan results, we'll be in the mood to celebrate."

17

OUTTA HERE

At the end of November came the third round of chemo, and three weeks later came the fourth. In this wintry, gray season, one month blurred into the next. I had entered the fog of cancer treatment. To make it worse, I had an unshakable cold. I dozed, in and out of sleep, expecting a call from Dr. Schuster's nurse practitioner, Danielle Land, who'd informed me at yesterday's appointment that this week's scheduled PET-scan had been postponed until December 29. She'd explained that inflammation from a cold, not to mention the inflammation from surgery, showed up in the recent CAT-scan and there was no telling cancer from, say, a sinus infection. In fact, she'd called Dr. Pochettino to get his take on the radiologist's report, which identified "a growing nodule, likely to be lymphoma"—a startling fact she mentioned as casually as an afterthought.

When she saw my stunned reaction, she reassured me that Dr. Schuster would be as unfazed by the finding as she was. Radiologists, she said, tend to err toward the worst, not infrequently offering alarming conclusions, lest they be accused of having missed something, whereas the treating doctors often interpret these images in a much more favorable light. "Honestly, I wasn't even going to mention it to you, and I probably shouldn't have until Dr. Schuster takes a look." She smiled cheerfully. "Stay healthy for the next three weeks so we can finally get a good PET-scan! I'll call you tomorrow as soon as I know anything."

In a congested haze, I anxiously awaited her call. When I woke from an afternoon nap in my bedroom, I first checked my phone—no missed calls—and then, on the way to the bathroom, I went down—dropped. In an instant it was lights out, legs vanishing from under me, and boom—black nothingness. When I came to, seconds later, I was on the floor, cheek on the carpet, as if I'd been napping there for hours. My head had fallen precariously close to the corner of the dresser; give or take an inch, we could have been facing questions about not only fainting but internal bleeding. *This can't be par for the course,* I thought.

When I climbed back into bed, I called my new primary doctor at Penn, Katie Margo, who promptly canceled another appointment and arranged to see me pronto. I went to the hospital, and within an hour she examined and diagnosed me. A sinus infection, after all. Sudafed was added to my daily cocktail.

Back home, my dad called to investigate his theory that my symptoms were being aggravated by the low barometric pressure. Dr. Schuster had assured me it was the prednisone, not blood backing up due to clotting, that was causing the "egghead effect"—this bloated feeling, aggravated by my seemingly chronic sinus infection.

The hours of the day dwindling, I sat with my laptop in my green chair. The Sudafed seemed to be making space in my head for creative thoughts, or at least for tiny sparks that flared up and dissolved. I'd begun to write notes about the experiences I'd had since August, for now recording only the clinical details I figured I wouldn't want to forget, if only for future healthcare purposes. I didn't dare to imagine I might one day use these recollections for artistic purposes.

I'd also been looking over drafts of other projects that had gone untouched for months and pretended to make progress. I was fascinated by my long hiatus from creative work, during which time

I'd wanted only to gaze at the clouds and trees, not to write about them or even to record my thoughts inspired by them. I'd recognized that it was a time to experience fully what I might otherwise be trying to capture in art. I'd recognized the floating away of that noble artistic impulse and found myself content to be, and to think, only in and of the moment.

As my living room grew dim, I checked for missed calls or texts from Danielle. I checked my email.

Instead, an email had come from Matt, in Nashville, with an attached jpeg of a new song he'd recorded called "Outta Here." He explained that the lyrics were inspired by the day he'd visited me in the hospital, during that long stretch when only time would tell if I'd need a stent to keep my graft from closing. *Elevator doors and exit signs . . . They're gonna taunt you till you wanna cry.* I was shocked by the beauty of the song, and, more so, by the notion that my friend had been so moved by our shared experience that he'd made music from it. I remembered the day, in that shadowy room, in a bed, a square of gray daylight visible through the white curtain. *Out the window tall buildings and a clear blue sky . . . High tops on the wire gotta be some kind of sign.*

Matt's voice rumbled out of the laptop speakers and through my veins, hitting the true note between terror and exuberance. *Get me outta here . . . I got nothin' to fear.* The thrumming guitar railed against the ache of the lyrics. I remembered feeling that day as if I were at a still point in the universe, sitting on a chair in my room, while others— family, friends, doctors—buzzed about. *Taking calls down by the Coke machine light,* out in the hallway or outside the building or miles away in their homes and offices, protecting me from their fears. *And the folks on the phone saying you'll be fine . . . Wait a minute are you sure they got this right . . . You couldn't see this comin' even if you tried.* I was at that still point again, staring out the window of my home, past bare trees, at the same gray sky. *Get me outta here . . . Get me outta here . . . Got nothin' to fear . . . Got nothin' to fear . . .*

I told Matt I was claiming the song as my personal anthem. Before the sun went down, I donned my headphones, cranked up the volume on my long walk to the corner, and wondered at this poetry and friendship, which, intertwined, had the power to transport me. *And someday soon . . . We'll sort it all out . . . How all of a sudden . . . Everything went south.*

18

TESTOSTERONE

Days before Christmas, Alex emailed a half dozen of us a *New York Times* article entitled "Are We Not Man Enough?" In the article, Steve Kettmann reports on Barry Bonds's conviction for obstruction of justice, which, "stemmed in part from his use of a testosterone-based balm famously known as 'the cream.'" Kettmann says "that in the more than eight years since Mr. Bonds was first accused of using performance-enhancing drugs, something strange has happened—millions of men have started to use the cream, too—or one of any number of similar treatments to make themselves look and feel younger and stronger."

I was intrigued less by the article than by the fact that I'd been included as a recipient of this email. I couldn't help wondering if I was being advised facetiously to use "the cream" as a supplement to chemo, or if I'd just been politely, or absentmindedly, included in this discussion on a topic about which I had very little to offer. "Extra testosterone does a lot for the body," Kettmann reports, "but it also gives an athlete a feeling of being unstoppable, of having an edge, of feeling, well, sexy."

My friends, on the other hand, were eager to opine on the matter, reveling in their healthy lifestyles, some explaining how they indulged in red wine, red meat, roller hockey, and women, others how they'd given up booze and beef, in exchange for roughage, rock climbing, and long runs.

My own absence from the exchange began to feel conspicuous, and I wanted to chime in, maybe with a joke about the stimulating effects of chemotherapy, before someone else broke the ice, perhaps by asking me what I thought about all this.

The conversation took an intimate turn when the oldest of the group confessed he'd resorted to "the cream" after a series of devastating blows—loss of his job, death of his father, demise of his marriage. Now he was once again his hard-charging, type-A, optimistic, passionate self. He said he'd gone to an endocrinologist, who, after diagnosing him as having low testosterone, prescribed a gel, to be lathered on every morning wherever his T-shirt would cover. After one day of use, he decided to try a more naturalistic approach to boosting testosterone—two fish oil pills and a vitamin D supplement in the morning and again at night; an increase in the intake of good fats, like almonds, walnuts, avocados, etc.; more "manly" workouts, with weights rather than running, or a combo of running with "muscle" exercises; more sex, porn, and self-satisfaction; better sleep; eating more red meat—preferably grass-fed.

At this point, I felt not just like an outcast, but like a member of a different species, so far removed from this world of the living that when John Bon next replied, I welcomed his exaggeration, laughing delightedly at his self-mocking bravado—until I realized he wasn't kidding: *I don't eat meat. I don't drink. I don't smoke. I don't do drugs. I have a fast motorbike and want a faster one. Sex twice a day for the last two years leaves me edgy—3-4 times makes me sleep better. Getting comfortable dropping in on head-and-a-half-high waves. Run 12+ miles coupla times a week for a laugh. Climbing harder than I've ever climbed before. Reading some Bukowski to keep the brain engaged. Good, clean livin'...*

What was I to make of this? And how should I reply? These

friends were caricatures of vitality, while I was a slug, who'd lost all sense of how his current condition may be skewing his perception of reality. *Sex twice a day for the last two years?* I didn't need chemo to find this enviable—*seriously?* Was John Bon's lifestyle the result of the pendulum-swing effect on a man who, after getting married and living in France for a decade, got a divorce and moved to Venice Beach, California? He certainly had no need for "the cream."

In the article, Kettmann concludes by asking, "Do we really want to feed a business culture that increasingly elevates cocksure confidence and pushiness above all else, especially if it filters into everyday life? In an era marked by the dangerous decisions of an entire industry full of gung-ho alpha males, shouldn't we be wary of a culture that pushes us even further in that direction? Maybe some quiet time for reflection or awareness of the consequences of one's actions might not be so bad—even if it means a little lower T."

There was no mistaking Alex's mocking irony, which restored my sense of reality. *I don't eat meat unless it's attached to a woman. Unbridled farting is important. Sex, post-modern philosophy, movies, loud live music, hiking and biking, a cocktail with fresh ingredients is essential. Drugs, too. We are all too rational. It's a dangerous thing. The occasional break is essential, and I'm not talking about a runner's high. I would recommend brushing your teeth with the gel. Gums are sensitive to things like that. Twice a day. And make sure to get the back molars.*

When I laughed, a voice stirred in me, hot-wired. Alex's wit had, not for the first time, jumpstarted my creative impulses. By now the winter sun had set, and the room had darkened. Mine was not your usual brand of cabin fever. I imagined that my beloved, healthy friends must be wondering if I'd been reading their emails all day. I had been fermenting. I was breaking down; I was effervescing. I started rolling in.

I'm all about drugs these days. Rituxan, Adriamycin, whole bags of it, right into the vein, bitches. 100 milligrams of prednisone, four days in a row, really gets my blood pumping, the muscles jacked—

Barry Bonds has got nothing on my swollen neck, venous congestion be damned. 10 milligrams of Coumadin to keep the blood thin, good and resistant to coagulation, because fuck clotting. Zofran for nausea, throw in some Ativan if I'm feeling hopped up, or if I'm really feeling nasty I make it a Marinol (as in legalize it, motherfuckers, and this is Pennsylvania, not Venice Beach). The metoprolol keeps the blood pressure low, lowers the heart rate, increasing the chances I'll faint (twice in the last month!), which is quite the adventure, let me tell you, especially if you're near a blunt object like the edge of my bedroom dresser and you're a serious bleed risk (whoah, where am I? Oh, I'm on the fucking floor! Holy shit, I fainted on my way to take a piss!). Aspirin. Vitamin C, zinc, to fend off the colds, but I've got my amoxicillin, which I've tapped for two full ten-day courses in the last six weeks, thanks to dizzying sinus and lower bronchial infections that have created virtual oceans of waves crashing in my head for week-long trips. Colace or Dulcolax, or any generic stool softener will do, morning and night, to keep it smooth, gentle, and predictable, as advertised! Believe me, all this poison stiffens things up, and you do not know constipation until you have had to take creative, self-stimulating measures to avoid an ER visit for an enema, not to mention a kind of bleeding that would undermine the purpose of all that Coumadin (this is not the kind of bleeding we're trying to prevent!). Prunes help too. I resisted, but, really, prunes.

Ten hours of sleep is sufficient. Maybe an afternoon nap. Most of the day I'm in my new state-of-the-art chair, easy to recline, but ideally comfortable in the upright position. I recommend the laptop pillow by Brookstone, solid surface, absorbs the heat. I can go six hours without blinking, maybe pause for a mid-afternoon Zofran. Tea twice a day. I drink water like a drain. Soup. Bread. Yogurt. I try to get outside once a day. I walk around the block, track the progress of the Barnes Museum going up on the corner down on the Parkway. If I'm feeling extra strong, I'll push it down to the far corner, not all the way to the museum on the hill, but right up to where the traffic turns, and then I bring it straight back home; it's a straight shot, right down the newly installed sidewalks, under the canopy of trees. If I need a rest, I'll park it for a few minutes on a bench at the Rodin Museum. Last week I walked all the way back from the anti-coagulation clinic—in West Philly—that's past the train station, over the bridge, and ten blocks to the Art Museum area. I wash my hands like I've got OCD (no more colds! at least until the PET-scan on the 29th), and I'm upping the skin cream use because we don't want to have to stanch the bleeding from cracked fingertips.

If I've got the appetite, I eat meat, all I can get my hands on. I eat fruit and vegetables (not too much green, because the vitamin K will offset the Coumadin), and soup and pasta and whatever the fuck I feel like, and I can't fucking wait to eat sushi again; I dream of sushi; I have reservations at Morimoto for Valentine's Day, which falls three weeks after my last scheduled chemo treatment, just in time to eat all the potentially contaminated, infection-inducing food I want, starting with raw fish. Otherwise I'm avoiding restaurant food and unwrapped food, for fear of bacteria, at least during the 5-10-day neutropenic stage (when the white blood cell count crashes, along with the immune system). Two weeks ago, during my "good week," I took my doctor friend Dan to Capital Grille and ate a 24-ounce porterhouse, the wedge salad with bleu cheese dressing, mashed potatoes and sauteed mushrooms. And a beer. My last blood test, which ran the gamut, showed I have a 150 cholesterol level. Low! In fact, the results of that test came the day of the Capital Grille dinner. When my doctor called with the results, I told her my plans for the evening and she told me to enjoy my steak. I made a toast to my cholesterol. My cholesterol level kicks ass.

The last CAT-scan showed the graft in my chest possibly narrowing further because of progressive scarring, which means my vascular system must form collateral veins and provide compensation and relief before the graft closes up. Go, collaterals! Seriously, fucking go, for godsake!!! In the meantime, I have days when I have to rest after playing Mr. Potatohead with my kid. I was cleaning my room the other day and found a pair of brand new running sneakers I bought in August. I can't wait to wear them, to walk past the corner that leads to the Art Museum, and then to run past it and then all the way down to Falls Bridge and around the eight-mile loop, which was my summer goal that got cut short.

One man's marathon is another man's walk around the block; one man's abstinence, another man's orgasm; one man's fast, another man's feast; one man's balance, another man's addiction.

Whatever: enjoy every morsel, gentlemen.

Here's to good health.

Minutes later their replies came in. I felt satiated, my muses pleased. I reclined in my green chair.

This must be the beginning of your next book, was the consensus.

My heart swelled.

If only this were fiction.

19

MERRY CHRISTMAS AND HAPPY NEW YEAR

For Christmas we went home to my sister Sue's house in Lancaster. I was so tired at the dinner table that I limped upstairs, crawled onto the nearest bed, and sank into pillows and the darkness of deep sleep. When I woke hours later, I felt warm and washed out.

Vana took my temperature, which was 100. We understood that, if my temperature hit 100.4, I was in danger of developing a life-threatening infection because of neutropenia. When the white blood cell count plummets, particularly the neutrophils—the body's precious infection fighters—the disarmed immune system can't fend off a simple virus. Numerous doctors and nurses had made the danger of neutropenia incandescently clear to me; if you get an infection, you have nothing to fight it off. Sepsis is a killer. There is no such treatment as a neutrophil infusion; the levels return to normal only on their own. In the meantime, the body requires precautionary IV antibiotics to guard against the threat of even the common cold.

As Vana escorted me downstairs, back to the festivities at hand, my head was in the stars, but somehow also felt filled with lead. I imagined my white blood cells vanishing like bubbles popping in the summer air—floating there, waxy, kaleidoscopic, and then gone.

When I awoke the next morning at my parents' house, the

strange stiffness I'd been feeling in my mouth had turned ulcerous. My temperature hovered at 100 until the afternoon, when it hit 101. I called Dan Landsburg, who'd given me his cell phone number in case of emergency. He advised that I go directly to the local ER to be admitted for IV antibiotics, reminding me that you don't play around with neutropenia. My dad didn't want me spending Christmas weekend alone in a room at Lancaster General Hospital. Instead, he drove me to the nearby outpatient clinic to get my blood checked.

My white blood cell count was 1300, my neutrophil count 5 percent—alarmingly low numbers—which explained why it felt as though a five-gram weight hung by a thread from every cell in my body. Despite the results, my dad was not convinced I needed to be admitted for IV antibiotics; instead, we stopped at the Rite-Aid on the way home to get Valtrex for my "herpes"—or, as Dad said (and I preferred), my "herpetic ulcers"—caused by a virus that could be treated with medication. He called Dan and persuaded him that the Valtrex would take care of the herpes and thus the fever. I had put my full faith in my father's care, and now, apparently, so had Dan.

When my fever was gone the next morning, it seemed my dad had been right. To be sure, we returned to the clinic to repeat the blood tests, which revealed an upward swing, with a total white blood cell count of 1,600 and 20 percent neutrophils. Still low, but I felt much better and so we agreed to stay the course. Mission accomplished; hometown hospital averted. I would be spending the holiday weekend convalescing in my parents' living room, monitoring my temperature and my swollen, aching cheeks. Merry Christmas.

• • •

Back in Philly three days later, I still looked like old Marlon Brando, the mouth ulcers bursting milky white at their growing centers. On the 29th, I went for my PET-scan, as planned. It was about time we got proof that the current chemo-cocktail was working.

In a small room I sat on a recliner behind a curtain. Glucose was administered intravenously and found its way throughout the body. The nurse apologized for the two Styrofoam cups of icy barium-colada she instructed me to drink, as if she were personally responsible for the foul-tasting stuff. I raised my cup, "Bottoms up!" and slugged the whipped metallic-coconut concoction that would help prime the body for the PET-scan's rays.

After the PET-scan, I went to schedule the follow-up appointment, when Dr. Schuster would review the test results. The post-Christmas schedules were full because of patients whose chemo treatments had been postponed for the holiday. So, my appointment wouldn't occur until January 5, which was also the date of my fifth chemo treatment.

When the day finally came, Vana and I braced ourselves in the examination room.

Dr. Schuster's smile relieved us when he entered. "After your treatment today, you'll get one more round of chemo at the end of the month—and then that will be that."

He explained that, despite the radiologist's reading of the recent CAT-scan, the so-called nodule did not appear to be "PET positive." He went to the computer at the corner desk and took the mouse from his assistant, who sat quietly before the keyboard. I could see that he was rereading my original pathology report, drawn toward the screen, newly intrigued by the case.

"Never saw this before," he uttered, the old familiar words, just loud enough for us to hear. "Been doing this thirty years, all over the world, never heard of lymphoma presenting in the vein wall like this."

As if we were just getting started.

He unlocked his gaze from the computer. "Definitely a case that should be written up." He gave his assistants an encouraging look. "Now's your chance."

I said, "Back in August Dr. Goren said he was going to write an article about it."

Dr. Schuster grinned ruefully. "The medical profession is terrible at continuity." He explained how doctors, especially at academic hospitals like Penn, where there's a constant influx of students and exodus of staff, don't have time to look backward. There was no time, for example, for those two young doctors back on Labor Day weekend to learn that it had not been a clot, but a malignant tumor obstructing my superior vena cava; no time for the doctors who treated me right here in this very institution to learn from my case, let alone doctors at other hospitals, right here in Philly or anywhere else in the world, who might one day treat patients with similar occlusions. A year from now, my dad would say, "That's why you're going to write about it."

Dr. Schuster stood, shook his head, then leaned back in toward the computer screen. "Good thing Pochettino got out all the tumor. Spared you the need for radiation."

"Why not spare me the chemo, too?" I asked, only half-facetiously.

He looked at me and smiled. "Forget what's in the books. Always get a doctor with gray hair. There's no substitute for experience." He presented his hand for me to shake. "Happy New Year."

• • •

In a week the neutropenic stage hit. I was so used to the dizzying symptoms that I almost didn't bother to check my temperature. When I checked at 5:30, it was 100.1. I emailed Danielle Land, who instantly replied, warning me to come to the ER if it hit 100.4. Come to think of it, she said, rush to the Perelman Center right now, before it closed at 6:00, so that I could avoid the ER and get my blood checked in the comfort of Dr. Schuster's office. But I couldn't even make it out the door by 6:00, much less hail a cab and get to Penn, so I decided to monitor my temperature and deal with the ER later if necessary.

I lay in bed while Vana cooked dinner, fed and bathed Nikitas, and put him to bed. When she poked her head in to check on me, I asked what was cooking, so delirious that I couldn't identify the smell of steak and fries, my favorite, which she'd whipped up in hopes of revitalizing me. The strategy worked. I went downstairs and devoured it all, sure I was on the mend. At bedtime my temperature was 100.2. I called my dad, who told me to take two Tylenol and get a good night's sleep.

I slept soundly despite sweating buckets. I'd been told not to worry about night sweats, typical of chemo patients. The next morning my temperature was 97.6, which I measured precisely with what seemed like newfound vision. It was only then, with my clearer perspective, that I realized I had been misreading the thermometer. What I thought had been 100.2 or slightly higher was actually between 100.4 or 100.5. I emailed Danielle to explain that I had been mistaking each notch on the thermometer for .1 degree, not .2 degrees. She instructed me to come immediately to the Perelman Center to get my blood work done.

Vana and I sat in the waiting room for three hours to get the results. Danielle appeared with a nervy smile, before turning her stern eyes on me. "You were definitely neutropenic yesterday and you should have been put on antibiotics right away." Her reprimanding glare turned relieved. "Last night you should have been admitted for emergency IV infusion." She took a deep breath, letting that sink in. "At this point, though, pill form will do."

"I'm an idiot," I said.

She reminded me of the morbid dangers of sepsis, then directed her attention to Vana, who surely appreciated the alarming gravity of the situation.

It suddenly occurred to me that I might have been neutropenic after every round of chemo and that I probably had fevers that had gone undetected, an easy mistake, I said, since the discomfort of fever would have been masked by the more overwhelming symptoms of total head congestion, coughing, and throat swelling, not to mention the Tylenol I popped to combat the headaches.

"Tylenol!" Danielle scolded. "You shouldn't be taking Tylenol!"

"Really? Uh-oh. But my dad—"

"It masks the neutropenic fever," she huffed. "And how do you misread a thermometer?"

"The notches, I—"

"You guys need a digital."

Vana said, "I bought one this morning."

Danielle fixed her eyes on me, smiling. "No more taking chances!"

I nodded.

"From now on Vana takes your temperature."

I figured I'd be fine reading the new digital job.

Later, when I told my dad about the whole regrettable episode, I was relieved to hear him say that, even if I'd read the thermometer correctly, he would have advised me just the same—take two Tylenol and get some sleep.

"You didn't seem so sick," he said, trusting his intuition, "certainly not as sick as you've been in the past."

"Well, that's for sure," I agreed, and we left it at that.

20

PREDNISONE

As much as I was looking forward to the sixth and final round of chemo, I was also dreading it. The weeks following my fifth treatment had whipped past with the usual nausea, malaise, and neutropenic lows. Now I was enjoying the good week, the third of three in the cycle, during which time I experienced a strange sense of peace while also bracing myself for the unpredictable emergence of an emotional beast that, my doctors assured me, was born of prednisone.

One afternoon I was hunched over in the dark pantry, growing irritated because I couldn't find a paper bag to deposit my empty ginger ale can for recycling, when Vana asked me how my day had been. My slight delay caused her to assume, reasonably, that I must be annoyed by the question. I stood upright, balancing myself against the doorframe. Blood flow returned to my head. Before I could reply, she observed, not quite gently enough for my liking at the moment, that I never complained about my physical condition.

My back was literally against the wall. She was giving me a look that felt more accusatory than inviting, though later she would claim that she'd truly meant to invite me to complain, to open up, to vent, etc. Of course, her observation that I *didn't* complain was, in my twisted view, a complaint in itself, one that I found infuriating not only for the obvious and unrecognized ironic fact that "You're *complaining* that I *never complain?!* You should be *praising* me for *not complaining!*" (These next complaints I kept to myself.) *You should be recognizing my positive attitude! Celebrating my stoic resilience! Throwing a party for my resistance to bitchiness! Organizing a parade for my aversion to griping! Adoring me for sparing you and the world any tiresome bellyaching! I'm happy to be alive, goddammit. Don't you see how happy I am? I don't have anything to complain about! You want me to whine about whatever discomfort I feel when I bend over? I'm alive! I'm just looking for a fucking paper bag to put this goddam can in!*

My irritability had evolved so slowly in the past few weeks, perhaps even months, that I'd barely noticed it consuming me, let alone manifesting itself in such monstrous form. I recognized my outbursts as outrageous expressions of my own impatience and frustration only after I'd unleashed them and Vana was left standing there, wondering at this strange beast who had replaced her husband.

She had returned to the tilapia frying on the stove. And then, just like that, I was sitting in my green chair, contemplating the matter. I thought, *Is this who I am? Who I've become? O prednisone! Be my scapegoat! Be the cause of this Jekyll and Hyde transformation, of this creature that feasts on those he loves. How I've grown accustomed to you, accepting your bloating presence, your cocaine-like kick that keeps me up at night. You infest my face like a nest of ants in my epidermis. You enter my blood and linger here.*

In charged moments like this, I remembered the incident in the hospital courtyard, when my mother and I stood outside the locked glass doors as the family walked past us inside. Since that day, I'd been reassured that prednisone was indeed the cause of such outbursts. My neighbor had told me that, when he was on prednisone in his twenties and thirties, he would date women and break up with them before any relationship developed because he could not tolerate their idiosyncrasies, even as he recognized his own unbearable impatience. He would spare them all, do the world a favor, and quarantine himself from it. An ex-student of mine, a battler of migraines and asthma, had said he spent a summer on prednisone, full of rage, straining to bottle up his emotions lest he lash out and recoil into a world of self-loathing, only increasing his depression. Hearing these stories, I felt lucky, even as my outbursts continued to torment Vana, who could hardly bear them any longer.

I called out to her from my green chair, "Sorry."

"It's okay," she generously lied. She turned off the stove.

"Just three more weeks," I told her.

She put on a smile. "Time for dinner."

Please don't give up on me now, I thought.

21

THINGS WE'RE LOOKING FORWARD TO

I was sitting on the toilet, leafing through the January issue of *Esquire*, when I came across a two-page spread announcing THINGS WE'RE LOOKING FORWARD TO IN 2012. I huffed, resisting the notion that anyone was looking forward to "Watching Pippa Middleton watch the London Olympics." Tiny, numbered photographs matched up with the extensive list of such "tiny pleasures" filling the bottoms of the pages. I wanted to dismiss it all as a shameless plug for upcoming products that publicists had managed to push on the magazine. But I couldn't help reading on. I became increasingly skeptical as I scanned the first column: "Beck's influence on Dwight Yoakam's new album," "The last of the *Twilight* movies," "Cheryl Strayed's gripping hiking memoir. That's right, gripping hiking memoir." And so on. Jennifer Lawrence in *The Hunger Games*. A new Oliver Stone flick. One World Trade Center tops out. Emma Stone in *The Amazing Spider-Man*. I thought, *Seriously? Are we really looking forward to Arnold Schwarzenegger's memoirs?*

Despite my cynicism, I felt a twinge of optimism, perhaps at the thought of a new Oliver Stone movie. But then, this optimism was tinged with another feeling I was not quite in touch with, feelings I recognized as my refusal to look forward to *anything* and my resentment towards anyone who might actually be looking forward to the iPhone 5. It wasn't that I had become a grouch, the present sour attitude notwithstanding. It was that I didn't presume anything about my future, about *a* future. I wouldn't let myself, or, I hadn't let myself—until now.

I was weeping in gleeful anticipation for Jonah Hill's *21 Jump Street,* certain I'd never watch this movie but confident I would at least exist on the planet when it came out in theaters, and right now the notion of sharing time and space with insignificant cultural phenomena seemed not just miraculous but positively heavenly. Sacha Baron Cohen playing a dictator in a movie loosely based on a novel by Saddam Hussein. This all seemed too good to be true, these things all impossibly glorious.

They'd saved the best for page two: Radiohead's new tour. Radiohead! Another Radiohead album! I was overwhelmed with joy. Another Batman movie. My joy was childlike Christmas-morning ecstasy. A new James Bond movie. *I would be alive to see this! Mad Men* was back! Are you kidding me? How close I had been to missing it all.

Arrested Development reprised.

Three Stooges reimagined.

Charlize Theron—

The opening of the Barnes Museum!

Yes, *Esquire* magazine had announced the momentous opening of the museum that was being erected a stone's throw from my front door. Vana and I would attend the grand opening with our premier membership. *Yes, we would!*

My own personal list spiraled from my mind: *Play golf with Chris. Walk the streets of New York with Lee. Catch Springsteen in South Philly with Rubin. Meet up with my writer buddies Bob and Marc at El Vez for nachos and bottles of beer and talk of fiction, journalism, and justice. Go to Nashville to visit Matt, hit the honky-tonks, and eat barbecue.*

Before any of these wishes materialized, Dr. Schuster would cheer us on at my first post-chemo appointment. "When are you guys going to start making babies again?" We'd chuckle nervously, and he'd assure us it was safe to procreate the old-fashioned way. No risk of poisoned supply, no reason to tap that frozen stock we'd stored just in case. At last, after treatment, Vana and I would fly to Florida to soak in the sun and release ourselves into our lives again, united, with blood flowing, bodies warmed, memories baked in, skin toughened.

When the sun shone in Philadelphia, I would go with Nikitas to the park. For now, we were confined to our small living room, but I was picturing the thawed fields down the street and the sandy beaches of Bethany, where soon we'd be throwing and running. Even if the blood backed up in my head and I was not fully mended, I was looking forward into what felt like eternity, where I was chasing my little boy in the grass or on the sand, and he was giggling over his shoulder, "I gotchu, I gotchu," and I was repeating, "I got *you*, I got *you*," and then I was wrestling him to the ground and by a miracle I was lifting him up with my arms toward the sun as he was saying, "Again, again."

With this glorious glimpse into the future came a kind of cracking open inside me, fortified walls giving way to an immense pressure, a rupturing then a gushing, and beyond the collapsing walls I saw the light of spring, which would be here soon, I understood. And now I believed *I will see spring,* an excruciatingly pleasing thought. I would be alive, or so I hoped and prayed, to be here to see—or not to see, if I so chose—Barbra Streisand and Seth Rogen on a cross-country road trip in *My Mother's Curse.*

22

QUARANTINE

At the end of January came the sixth and final round of chemo. The nausea hit hard in the first few days, and by day five my body began to weaken as the dreadful neutropenic stage set in. I decided to quarantine, to avoid contamination. I would stay in my bedroom, propped up against a stack of pillows in bed, watching Ken Burns's eleven-hour series *The Civil War*—the DVD boxed set I'd snagged from my sister's house at Christmas.

When Vana brought me meals, I set the plates on the bed and ate while watching the documentary on my laptop. At bedtime, Vana held Nikitas in her arms at the doorway. He reached out to me for a hug. "No, no," Vana said. "Say goodnight to Daddy." He waved and blew me kisses. When the coast was clear, I went downstairs for a snack or medicine. No more fainting or falling, I'd decided, keeping a firm hand on the dresser as I wound my way to the bathroom and back to bed, where I remained riveted.

My sudden passion for American history amazed Vana. I dozed off and returned to the battlefield, grainy black-and-whites floating on the screen and in my dreams. I couldn't understand why McClellan wouldn't act, wouldn't attack, after having assembled a Union army that so far outnumbered the South's. Lincoln must have been apoplectic hearing of McClellan's paralysis. And yet the wise old president wouldn't fire him. Meanwhile, the South had their way with the North in battle after battle, two years of virtual annihilation. McClellan left the scene, only to be rehired by Lincoln and only to repeat his most peculiar behavior—at one point failing to attack in a situation that might have won the war for the North and ended all the butchery. Lincoln went South, met with McClellan, perhaps because he needed to see all this hesitancy to believe it, and fired him once and for all.

Vana interrupted to say that this was hardly uplifting stuff, that I should watch *Sideways,* our old favorite. I said that right now a movie about a middle-aged, unpublished, divorced English teacher didn't hold quite the same comic appeal as it used to. Instead, these six discs, in well-measured doses, would get me through the neutropenic stage. I just needed to get over the hump. I could feel the inevitable wave of fatigue. I could only hope it wouldn't be accompanied by the confounded fever.

Meanwhile, Nikitas got a fever that spiked at 105, an unprecedented high. Vana considered taking him to the ER, but on my dad's advice treated him with Tylenol and by morning his temperature was back to normal. My mom arrived to help so that Vana could go to work. Nikitas stayed home from day care. I stayed sealed up behind my closed door. At night Nikitas's temperature hovered in the low 100s—out of the woods, my dad assured us.

On the ninth day post-chemo I slept soundly enough, until 3:30 a.m., when I woke and fought my pillows for an hour before wending my way to the bathroom. Back in bed, feeling fatigued to the core, I took my temperature. 100.6. High. *Too high.* I didn't want to go to the emergency room any more than Vana did. I took my temperature again. 100.4. Still too high—the tipping point, the exact tenth of a degree that marked the neutropenic fever.

I began to get dressed.

"What are we doing?" Vana was awake.

"Going to the ER."

Quietly she got out from under the covers.

For the moment we remained not fully committed to such a venture, waiting for the other to offer a good reason not to leave home at this hour, so unpleasant was the prospect of returning to the hospital, just days, it seemed, before I might recover altogether and spread my wings, and we would all fly toward the sun and spring and blossoming flowers and all things happy.

Vana telephoned the hospital to inform the oncologist fellow on call that we were on our way. The operator said that she would page Dr. Schuster, who minutes later called my cell phone. "Good morning," I said. I described my symptoms. He asked what treatment I was on. Sixth, I said. "Figures, last one," he said. "Oh, well, it's almost over. We have to find out if you're neutropenic, and if you're not, they'll just send you home."

My gut told me I'd be staying—a baseless hunch I kept to myself.

"Poetic, really," I said to Vana.

"Oh, yes," she said, with an ironic flair. "It's the perfect bookend— to begin and end at the ER." She laughed.

I nodded. "Very nice."

"The perfect *arc* to the story," she said, indulging me with the kind of aesthetic observation she believed I must be sparing her.

I smiled, surprised by this cheerful cooperation, feigned as it was.

My mother entered the hallway from the guest room, where she'd been sleeping on the futon. It was by luck she was here tonight. We told her our plans. "Don't worry about things here. He'll be fine," she assured Vana, whose eyes were on Nikitas's closed door. In her nightgown, my mom followed us downstairs. Teary eyes belied her composure. She was too used to seeing me setting out for the hospital. Only this time I hadn't packed a bag. At the door I hugged her and told her, "I'll be all right—back soon," and for no good reason I believed it.

• • •

In the empty ER waiting room, the TV weatherman reported unseasonably high temperatures for the upcoming days—summer weather, highs in the sixties. Nurses worked casually at their desks. I was swiftly escorted to a room, where I climbed onto the stretcher and a nurse drew my blood. My temperature had dropped to 100.2. Vana and I shared relieved yet rueful grins. Had we waited an hour— or had I not awakened to use the bathroom—we wouldn't be here right now.

By 6:00 a.m. my temperature was 99.5, and by 8:00 it was 98.6.

I felt euphorically drained, eager to head home.

The returning test results showed my white cell count to be .6, raising the eyebrows of the doctors and nurses. The neutrophil count was zero—*zero* infection-fighting white blood cells.

"In the lab, that gets a red test tube," a nurse said. "Not good."

She reminded me that with an infection, and without antibiotics, I could become septic and die. Immediately, blood cultures were taken, infections investigated.

I considered the pros and cons of being kept in this ER room, just outside which contagion and bacteria-spreading patients floated by on foot and on stretchers. A woman across the hall screamed, "Well, then, fuck you, Jesus!" Evidently, the doctors, nurses, and security staff were too much for her resistance. "I want my children! Don't take my children!" Whatever her ailment, it was of such grave concern that these professionals were determined to subdue her in the face of her violent, hysterical protests. Minutes later a calm settled over the wing. Vana sat on a chair next to the sliding glass door that refused to shut all the way. A stern motherly voice reminded the patient, "Now you have to lie there and try to relax," and just then the woman flew from her restraints, cursing frantically. She darted out of the room and down the hallway, where security guards and doctors apprehended her and returned her to her room, this time sedating her and securing her to her bed with restraints.

White coats whipped past, blue scrubs lunging. Quiet again, she slept, if you could call it that, for hours, her face visible beyond the broad shoulders of a red-haired nurse or orderly, who sat in a chair in the doorway, chatting with other nurses and orderlies about their jobs and which shifts they liked best.

"It's overtime," one said. "Ain't like I'd be doing anything else at four-thirty in the morning."

• • •

Vana and I dozed as the antibiotic entered my vein. I'd been told I was soon going to be transported to Rhoads, the luxurious oncology unit where I'd stayed in October. But now hours had passed without a visit from anyone.

When a nurse dropped by to ask if we had any questions or requests, we reminded her that I was a cancer patient with no functioning immune system, being held in the ER, where contagious patients were loitering in the hallways and the door wouldn't stay shut. She said that a private room might not be available today, that there was an overflow of ER patients waiting for admission, and that discharges occurred in the afternoon and often rooms didn't open up until dinner time. "I'm giving you the real story," she said. "I'm not saying people are liars. I'm just saying they might tell you what you want to hear. You hungry?" She left and returned with two boxes of cereal, Raisin Bran and Cheerios, and a small container of milk.

We thanked her for her kindness and honesty.

"Hang in there," she said.

• • •

In the dark, dozing, Vana and I caught a news story of a massive car accident in the South, where a strange cloud system prevented the accident's initial smoke from dissipating. Instead, it collected on the earth's surface, blinding drivers. Among the fatalities was a family of parents and their children, except for one daughter, a lovely teenage girl, who survived the crash.

"There's no point in going on after that," Vana said, "after losing everything."

I wasn't sure where she was going with such a comment, or where she expected me to take it. My thinking about the girl and her grim situation was obviously different from Vana's. I was rooting for the girl in the face of her misery and sorrow. I bit my tongue, not wanting to sound unsympathetic or, worse, inadequately committed to those I love.

After a moment I couldn't help myself. "She didn't lose *everything*. You just go on."

Vana gave me a grave look. I got the message: *why must you challenge everything?*

I shrugged, half-embarrassed. And then, "What about Holocaust survivors? How should any of those people go on? Can you imagine a Holocaust survivor killing himself? No way."

Vana scrunched her face at my outrageous analogy. "Don't you understand? It's just a way of expressing empathy."

"I get it." I spared Vana the philosophical dialogue unfolding in my mind. Then I said, "If I die, you go on, damn it. Because I love you. I want you to live."

She humored me with a sour grin. "Okay, honey."

"Okay," I said, with finality, as if I'd nudged her toward a brighter vision of life.

• • •

Vana went home to take a shower and returned a few hours later. "No fever," she reported. Nikitas was on the mend. I remained on my gurney, despite the promise of a real bed. In Vana's absence,

I watched two episodes of *CSI* or some such show featuring cops going after inventive sexual predators. Then CNN, enduring more talk of Romney versus Newt and the virtues of negative campaign ads. Once again, I dozed.

At four in the morning Vana was long gone and I wished I had packed a bag after all or at least brought a book, but it had seemed like bad karma to come so well prepared. When she returned in the morning, she was shocked to see I was still laid up in the same room. She delivered a bag of clothes, along with Bill Bryson's *A Walk in the Woods*, ginger chews, an orange, and an egg-and-cheese sandwich, "made with love," she said, so I ate it promptly.

By mid-afternoon of day two in the ER, the nurse said I probably wouldn't get a room again today, discharges were not scheduled, and I was far from first in line. I joked with Vana about sneaking out with her or catching a cab on my own in a few hours. The nurse chimed in, "You've made it this far. No sense in screwing up now. Your numbers are still low."

After Vana left for the day, I couldn't muster the energy to read Bryson's book, much as I was drawn by the thought of getting lost in someone else's unfortunate adventure. I ate the lunch that arrived on a tray—turkey and beans—and snacked on ginger chews. I napped and watched TV, resigned to spend the night right where I was, on my gurney, hoping for a little help from Ativan. By eleven, I was watching Jon Stewart, but I didn't make it to the first commercial. No one had bothered to tell me that there were no rooms available after all.

• • •

On day three, a team of young oncologists entered the room to discuss my prognosis. They apologized that I was still in the same unpleasant place, still on the IV antibiotic.

I squirmed, wearing the jeans, sweater, socks and boots I'd arrived in, trying to get comfortable on the gurney, my lower back pulsating with pain. I cracked more jokes, less jokingly, about calling a cab.

"Keep the door shut and you'll be fine," was the encouraging message. "You did the right thing coming here."

My white blood cell count from the morning's test was 1.7, a nice leap, but far from sufficient to free me to catch the next cab.

"That's a great book, isn't it?" one of the doctors said. "That's the *one* book I read in high school that I remember. I would laugh out loud in class."

I managed a smile. "I love it." I didn't mention that in another life I might have been his teacher.

After they left, I ate my breakfast. I read for a while. I ate my lunch.

At last, the nurse poked her head in. "They have a room for you, so get your stuff ready."

There wasn't much to assemble. By four o'clock, the man who'd checked my vitals the day before announced, "All right, my man, I'm taking you to your room."

On the way out of the ER, approaching the elevators, I said, "Stop! I want to say hi—" I pointed to the doctor facing a computer screen, beyond a crowd. I couldn't remember her name, but I'd never forget that moment, her face pinched tenderly with regret, her sorrowful words. *"This could be fatal . . ."* I was wheeled around the counter to an opening. She turned to face me, this pale stranger wearing a mask and hat, both of which I promptly removed.

"Do you remember me?" I asked.

She rose from her chair and approached. "Yes, I do. Whatever happened to you?"

I told her the story, how I'd spent four days here that first time; returned a week later; got surgery to remove that mysterious blockage, which turned out to be lymphoma; just finished chemo; back here now with a bout of neutropenia.

She shook her head in wonder.

"I was hoping to see you—*Dr. Utley*," I remembered. "I wanted to thank you for taking care of me that night."

She said she was so glad to hear of my progress and wished me well.

On the long stretcher ride to Rhoads, my charming driver told me that the doctor I'd just thanked had started her job here in mid-August. He said, "That would have been one of her first nights—maybe her first."

I was amazed at the thought of what it must have been like for her, telling me that I wouldn't be making it to the Phillies game, and then later that I might not be making it out of here alive. She made me believe we were in it together.

"How you feeling now?" the orderly asked.

"Clear PET-scan," I said. "Fever's down but the white blood cell count is low. My wife is back and forth between me and our son. He just had a 105 fever, but he's better now."

"A few days ago my niece had a 106 or 107."

"Wow." I figured he had the facts wrong, or he was exaggerating.

"Her aunt went to her in the morning and found her blue. She was unconscious till the doctors at the hospital revived her and got her temperature down. Saved her life."

I shook my head. "Unbelievable." I was ashamed I'd doubted him.

He dropped me off and wished me well.

I nodded. "Thank you."

In my room I kept thinking that at any given moment we are all within one or two degrees of separation from someone who is going through some great suffering worse than our own. One question leads to the next, and suddenly the orderly is telling you about his niece's deadly fever; or the cab driver, just last week, is telling you about his wife's cancer, how the doctors botched the surgery, how he was walking with her to the opera when she first felt the pain, how a week later she was dead. And there you are, with your cancer, chatting it up with the driver, in the back seat of this cab, like the ones you've been in a thousand times before but always sitting in silence or chatting about the weather or traffic. But now other topics spring up, and this man's telling you his story because it's obvious that you really are interested, not because you have cancer, which you haven't mentioned, but because it feels natural and good to be sharing in his loss. You tell him you're sorry, and you wish each other well, and when you get out of the cab, life is richer, cab rides are no longer the same, nothing is, and everyone you see you understand is alone and in pain, or they have been, or they will be, but the realization doesn't make you sad—it makes you feel more alive.

• • •

The window in Rhoads 614 overlooked the rooftops of the Penn campus, purple-green metal awnings and pointed domes, brick facades and concrete window sashes, small arched windows lined with thick silver seams. Just out of view was the promenade where, months ago, I dragged my IV pole and met Vana and Nikitas, sat on a bench and watched him walk and fall, dig in the dirt, throw stones.

How was it that I had only fond memories of this place? Even those moments that had been filled with the deepest fear were marked by some expression of love I recalled with gratitude.

The young doctor who had liked *only* the Bryson book in high school popped his head in to ask if I was pleased with my room, as if there were any doubt.

"Almost finished." I flashed my paperback, whose cover featured a bear mugging for the camera before a backdrop of lime-green leaves.

He gave me a thumbs-up. "Good work."

The sun was beginning to set beyond campus, a thin stroke of orange blending with pink hues on the horizon, the skies streaked with white clouds dimming. The room had lifted my spirits and I was in no hurry to go home.

Vana visited for a few hours. Nikitas was just getting over his fever, so she told me to take my time returning home. She sat in the padded nook by the windows, and I sat in my recliner. We held hands and stared at the sunset and the sky that filled the window. I teased her about doing it in the bathroom, and then we made our way in there, hugging and kissing, happy to feel stabilized in each other's arms.

After she left, I was back into Bryson's book, as he neared the end of his long walk in the wilderness. I finished in time to catch Jon Stewart. The nurse got the antibiotic going and in the middle of the night slipped in to detach the tube from the port in my arm. I was in a haze while the phlebotomist drew my blood at 6:00 a.m., and by the time I awoke I was told my white blood cell count was 7.4, a higher number than I could remember ever having. Team Oncology arrived and the doctor who'd been running the show said we would forgo the morning's antibiotic—I was off the IV—and if I didn't get a fever between now and dinner time, I could go home by early evening.

I climbed out of bed, opened the shade, and dared to think of this milestone as being the beginning of the end, or just the beginning.

The next day, Vana got sick. A cold, but bad—fever, chills, the full catastrophe. She'd been keeping it all at bay, biding her time, until the rest of us were taken care of.

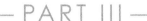

That a marriage ends is less than ideal; but all things end under heaven, and if temporality is held to be invalidating, then nothing real succeeds.

—John Updike

The truth will set you free. But not until it is finished with you.

—David Foster Wallace, *Infinite Jest*

23

HEAVEN ON EARTH

G ardens of dirt formed the perimeter of the Barnes Museum construction site. Sidewalks around a chain link fence still guarded its borders. I deeply inhaled the February air, which to me was cold, though it was fifty degrees and a group of girls were wearing sweaters with sleeves rucked up to the elbows. In hat and gloves, coat, and scarf, I took aim on the distant mark, the splash of blue sky and blacktop of the Parkway beyond the long sidewalk, now immaculately straight after renovation, the whole spectacle receding in dramatic symmetry like an optometrist's exam or a DaVinci drawing.

As I passed the Barnes's front yard and entered the Rodin's expanse of sprawling green on the next block, I was overcome with the revelation that I was feeling well, and that this sensation might be sustained—that illness might soon be behind me and I might grow stronger each day. I took in gulps of air as tears streamed. In a clearing in the trees, I saw the steps of the Art Museum, where black specks, weekenders strolling, flecked the concrete in the far distance. I was determined to make my way to the top. I felt like a lost wanderer at the fuzzy edges of home, where I'd been hovering for eons, never truly thinking I would return.

Steadying myself, I passed The Thinker and George Washington and the Native Americans and caribou and moose and kids climbing this gigantic sculpture of our country's patriarch crossing the Delaware. I approached the soft-pretzel peddler and the T-shirt man by the Rocky sculpture—and then those immortal steps. I took my time climbing. In no hurry, I celebrated each step. At the top, beyond the fountains and vast plateau, between the columns, hung blue banners, each with one white letter, spelling out VAN GOGH. I imagined a blank canvas on a wall in a garage converted into a studio in some future house I hoped to live in, somewhere not far outside the city. When I turned to take in the view, the city appeared both remote and familiar, and I felt at home.

With this satisfying thought came the urge to keep venturing out, so days later I took the train to Lancaster to see my nephew, Niki, play in his last home game, where they were honoring the seniors and their parents. On the train I felt like an adventurer, the kind of person who climbed mountains, hiked treacherous trails. My dad picked me up at the station. I'd told him I wanted to surprise Sue at her house—her sick brother trekking home to see her son's game.

When I arrived in Sue's kitchen, she led me giddily to a chair, then brought me one delectable dish after another, which I devoured—a bowl of *avgolemono* soup, a meatball sandwich, on and on. In minutes my great adventure came to a gut-wrenching halt. I had a stomachache, like the one I'd had nights earlier, clutching my knees to my chest until the pain subsided hours later.

My dad explained that this sensation came from the stomach muscle contracting from acid buildup. For months I'd been taking Zantac for nausea, so it made sense that there would be flux once I tried to get off the drug. On the way to the game, we stopped at a mini market, where my dad ran in to get Zantac and a bottle of water. We drove to my old high school and sat in the parking lot, waiting for the drug to take effect. The newly erected gym reminded me of decades gone by. In a half-hour I felt relief.

We entered just as the seniors were walking with their parents to center court. Niki spotted me gripping the railing, on the upstairs track that ringed the bleachers. He nudged his friend and pointed to his Uncle Jim. The friend squinted, puzzled, then recognized me. I waved, happy to be home, though I was a stranger now.

I sat next to Sue, who proudly introduced me to her friends. I used to be the brother who'd written the novel. Now I was the brother who'd gotten cancer and was obviously on chemo—pale-faced, bald, and bloated. And yet I felt triumphant, being here, the object of admiring, sympathetic smiles. But I also felt defeated, watching the game from inside a body that felt like a loaner, nostalgic for this place. Niki went on to score fourteen points in a nail-biter of a loss that kept his team out of the playoffs.

• • •

The next morning, I went with my dad to the local seminary, where once a month he got together for big-topic conversations with a group of about fifteen semi-retired septuagenarians like himself who relished the investigation of questions with no clear answers. This week's roundtable topic was heaven. The moderator, a good-humored, white-haired man reminded everyone of the assigned reading for today, and he welcomed debate. Dad jumped right in, cited the first beatitude—"blessed are the weak in spirit, for theirs is the kingdom of heaven"—and went on to explain the significance of the present tense, "Blessed *are* . . . Theirs *is* . . . " that heaven is here and now and it is those who are continually striving to know God—the weak in spirit—who are blessed.

I wanted to applaud. One attendee after another offered savvy insights. I was content to listen, in the shadowy corner of the chestnut-red room lined with aged bookshelves. But after some spirited discussion, the moderator insisted that no one should speak twice until everyone had spoken.

My hometown priest had arrived late and sat in a chair against the far wall. My dad had invited him to join the group months ago. When he was called on to speak, Father Alex proclaimed that heaven *must* exist, it just *has* to in order to justify the suffering that people endure on earth. All will be made right in heaven, he said. It is the only way to make sense of the inequality of human lives on earth. How else to explain how blessed *our* lives are, in contrast to the lives of those around the world who suffer from poverty, oppression, and other such horrible conditions?

I thought how pleasantly logical this theory was and how it presumed the existence of not only a just and loving God, which, of course, was a priest's reasonable presumption, but also a universe designed sensibly, with fairness in mind. I wondered at my own faith, which I could measure only by the amount of thought I devoted to trying to understand my own uncertainty.

Everyone else had spoken but me. All I could think to say was that I'd recently heard actor Jeff Bridges in an interview saying how he tries to "live like you're already dead, man . . ."

I couldn't begrudge the blank stares.

I said I believed I'd experienced "earth as it is in heaven" and how it seemed to me the transition from here to there should not be difficult, how I'd been right at the edge, where I felt myself already sliding from one realm to the other, and how, as I returned to "real life," it did not take long before that precious sense of heaven on earth became intermittent and fleeting, something to strive for, impossible to sustain.

A long silence followed, the stares thoughtful, a few sorrowful. Maybe they were contemplating the "edge" they were approaching, and wondering what existed on the other side. Or maybe they were wondering, as I was, if this was it, if earth was the only place to find heaven.

When the conversation ended, I was eager to leave. Out in the hallway, Dad suggested we ask Father Alex to join us at a diner for breakfast to continue this discussion before I headed back to Philly. He grinned. I agreed, like my father, forever striving to know. No matter what the future, or eternity, held for us, we would go to our graves more strongly bound to each other, father and son, weak in spirit, and blessed.

· · ·

The excruciating pain I experienced in Lancaster returned several times before an MRI revealed gallstones. The chief gastroenterologist at Penn prescribed rarely used pills in hopes of disintegrating them, determined to avoid surgery lest he cut into an unforeseeable collateral vein or lest the SVC clot during surgery. He gave me his business card in case of an emergency.

When another pain, in my groin this time, had me back at Penn, the surgeon who specialized in hernias lifted his nose from my extensive records and asked, "What did you do to deserve all this?"

I said, "What did I do to deserve to be spared?"

The doctor considered this question.

Then he said, "A strained muscle, most likely from overexertion on the stationary bike."

I welcomed the treatment plan—"Give it a rest."

24

ONCE MORE UNTO THE BREACH, DEAR FRIENDS

Three weeks post-chemo, instead of bracing myself for nausea, I was looking forward to Valentine's Day. First, Vana and I would go to the spa for massages. Then to the museum for the Van Gogh exhibit. Finally, to Morimoto for sushi. Today would be a celebration not only of our thriving, or surviving, romance, but also of eating raw fish without fear of bacterial infection.

I was becoming my own clinician, monitoring my symptoms, trying to understand the mysterious, dynamic world inside me, the variations and fluctuations beneath the healed wound, the fading scar as I inched my way back into the world of the living. There were times when the venous congestion felt like Chinese torture, the pressure intensifying, the blood rising at minuscule levels in my neck, in my face, up to my eyes, by the day, the hour, the minute. I wanted to believe that some of this discomfort might be only in my mind, that the sensations were normal. But when I twisted to reach into the thick sleeves of my coat, I couldn't deny the strained circulation, a feeling I would forever associate with the moment last August that extended into eternity. When I drove—turning the wheel, rotating the arms, twisting around to parallel park—I tried to accept with grace the sensations of blood flow ceasing, or threatening to cease, like a clutch of hands around the neck, a phantom strangler. Seconds later, the flow returned to normal—my new normal—whatever that was.

Dad called to ask how my symptoms were. He wasn't surprised when I told him I felt worse than yesterday. The barometric pressure was climbing, he reported hopefully, and reminded me of his theory of causation—that my symptoms were influenced by outside forces, including the weather. He predicted that when the sun came out, I'd be feeling more energetic. He explained that it was this same dynamic relationship, between the body and the climate, that allowed arthritics to predict rain.

By the time Vana and I got to the spa, my neck and head felt bloated. During the massage, I felt restored, but afterward, and for the rest of day, the blood seemed ready to rise to fill the balloon I imagined expanding from the center of my head and pressing at the backs of my cheekbones and eyes.

I was trying to stay optimistic. I reminded myself that it was a cold, gray day and that this was the most active I'd been since last summer, *So what can I expect?* The sun would come out—first literally, then figuratively.

· · ·

In March I was gearing up as if it were the first day of school, which for me it was. I'd decided to go to Penncrest to get a feel for the place, and a feel for myself in it, before I headed back for good. I wanted to see how it felt driving thirty minutes on I-95, walking into the building, talking with colleagues, being around the kids. I stayed out of the way of my substitute teacher, who had been there since September and seemed to be at home in my classroom, despite the surprising fact that she'd left my posters hanging on the wall and even my framed family photos sitting on the desk, for *six months.* "You should have removed these things," I said. Tenderly she looked at me and said, "This is your room."

In the cafeteria, I called out to the one student I knew, a girl who was the editor of the high school's literary magazine, for which I was faculty advisor. We'd swapped a few emails about the annual publication's floundering progress; she was eager for my return, hoping I might put a charge into the mission. But when she heard my voice, she turned vaguely in my direction and, seeing only a baldish stranger, turned back toward the friends she was talking to. I approached her, smiling, and said, "Hi." She beamed, embarrassed, attempting to disguise gracefully whatever other emotions she was feeling—*fascination? fear? sadness?*—but I felt welcomed. I was eager to return to this place, though it was not yet noon and I was already feeling whipped.

I would overlap with my substitute for three days before taking the reins. Teachers had heard I was back. They popped into my classroom or, when I walked past their rooms, slipped into the hallway, where they greeted me. Some mentioned "Mal," Mr. Malkovsky, the physics guru, who'd been out all year with pancreatic cancer. The news about Mal had been less hopeful than the news about me, they said, but not hopeless, as he endured more treatment and remained out. I thought about the seniors whom both Mal and I taught, or *would* have taught, these kids who'd had two teachers out with cancer. They must have thought, *What are the odds?*

I was not consciously nervous, being there, but all this talking, and even just *thinking* about talking, up there in front of those expectant faces next week, made the heart race. It had become clear that stress increased my symptoms, which made sense—internal pressure constricting the flow. I was always trying to breathe more easily, to keep my voice steady and quiet. The kids would think I was still sick or just the mellowest teacher they'd ever had, or heard, barely.

Back in the classroom, the students glanced at me politely, settling at their desks. Maybe I was pushing myself unnecessarily. Why not just stay home, rest, exercise, restore myself in peace and return to work in September? Some teacher friends had joked that I was nuts—why come back now? I didn't want to wait, only to return next fall, as if the whole year had never happened. I wanted to claim something of it. I wanted to be a part of it.

When the students filed in for a lazy last day with their long-term sub, snacking on chips and cupcakes and signing farewell cards, they smiled in my direction, welcoming me back for good in their quiet way. At first, I felt gun-shy, not yet ready to engage, but as the day wound down, I eased into the scene, as did the kids. We met somewhere in the middle. Some said how they'd been concerned for me, having heard about their sick teacher, or the man who would have been their teacher. Now here you are, they said. *Here I am.*

In the parking lot after school, I aimed my face at the warm sun. I was both exhausted and energized. I checked the barometric pressure. It was on the rise. Come Monday I would be back here for good.

• • •

On my dad's advice, and against my loyalties to Penn, I was driving to another well-known Philadelphia hospital to see Dr. Cliff Anders—coincidentally, an old colleague of Dr. Pochettino. My dad had been in contact with Dr. Anders and told him about my case. He'd also talked to several doctors about angioplasty, which they believed might be a real option at some point. Maybe I should ask Anders about angioplasty as well, Dad had said. I felt disloyal to Dr. Pochettino, especially when I'd called Penn's radiology department and asked them to send all my images to Dr. Anders.

Dad said Anders had worked with CorMatrix and had been doing cutting-edge stuff. He'd told me to make an appointment, just to feel Anders out, to see what he says about the recurring symptoms. "We might as well find out all we can," Dad said. "No big deal. Pochettino doesn't have to know. We're not exactly getting a second opinion. Maybe Anders will have some new ideas. Maybe he'll give us some insight about where we go from here, and how."

It was a brisk sunny day—the barometric pressure was high—
and I was feeling fine. I stopped at the nearby Starbucks and bought
a fruit smoothie and the new Springsteen CD, displayed next to the
graham crackers. On the car radio I kept hearing the same ad on
NPR about the new treatments being offered by Cancer Treatment
Centers of America and their state-of-the-art, minimally invasive
nano-knife, capable of doing biopsies in those hard-to-reach-places.
Too late, I thought, and wondered at the technology that would be
available a year from now, five years from now, picturing nano-bots
racing through the blood stream, collecting data. I popped in my new
CD and stepped on the gas, jamming "We Take Care of Our Own"
through the city, away from Penn.

In the waiting area, Dr. Anders asked if I was there to see him. I
said, "I'm Dr. Zervanos's son," and he gave me a puzzled look.

After a moment, he said, "You're the SVC guy. Pochettino's
patient. You hear he's going to Mayo?"

Mayo, as in Mayo Clinic? In Minnesota? Dr. Pochettino is leaving?

"No," I said. I must have appeared shaken.

Anders must have recognized in my reaction that this was not yet
news meant for public consumption—or at least not for Pochettino
patients.

"Wait here," he said, and walked away.

Minutes later he waved me back to his office, where his nurse
practitioner was at the computer, struggling to open my CAT-scan
files on the CDs I'd sent weeks earlier.

Anders was an easy six-four, two-forty, compact as an NFL tight
end. Afghan war vet memorabilia filled the shelves, along with mini-
American flags and a couple of floppy black Bibles, the malleable,
durable kind a soldier might take into combat. He shuffled some
papers at his desk. He said he'd just called Alberto—Pochettino.
He muttered something about having spoken too soon about his
leaving. Nothing was official. I imagined the phone call that had

just transpired, Alberto dressing down his old underling, who could never keep it under wraps, always too eager to be out in front.

"So, tell me what happened to you," Anders said. "Your version"—as if there were another version I knew.

He listened to my synopsis, while the CAT-scan CD sputtered on the screen behind him, the images a long way from downloaded. "Your dad is freaking out about the CorMatrix," he said. I tried not to take offense. My dad's emails, always copied to me, offered sober clinical descriptions of my case, scrupulously recounting my ordeal, in the interest of helping a fellow doctor. I figured Anders was trying to buddy up with me, by dissing my father—two young dudes having a laugh at the old man's expense—assuming I must be as perturbed by my dad's effort as he obviously was. He insisted that the narrowing of my SVC could have happened with any material, not just CorMatrix. It was just bad luck—and he wasn't just saying that because he was friends with Pochettino.

I wasn't sure whose interests he was trying to protect or why he thought I meant to undermine them. I offered an un-accusing stare that appeared to irritate him further. I said, "I'm on Coumadin," and explained that a stent had been considered but avoided in light of my stabilized symptoms and the promise of collateral veins.

He said, "You need a stent."

"A stent? I was just saying—"

"No question about it. I don't want to see you in my operating room with your head swollen due to a clot, and then we've really got a problem on our hands."

"I don't want to see that happen either. Why would I have a clot?"

"Because you'll have to go off Coumadin," he said.

"Why? When?"

"You don't want to be on Coumadin for the rest of your life. Believe me. There's a one-percent chance of a serious bleed on Coumadin. Every year, you have to figure you're facing a one-percent chance of a serious bleed."

"One percent? Is that so bad? What are the risks connected with having a stent?"

He grinned. "You're asking me to play God."

"No, I'm not."

He sighed. "Doctors have to make decisions sometimes based on knowledge and experience—not certainty."

"I understand that, but isn't it reasonable for me to want to compare the risk?"

He sneered. I was beginning to think he was taking my questions personally.

He said, "With Coumadin there are studies with reliable data. With stents in veins—extraordinary cases like yours—there are no such studies. You're in uncharted territory." His stare softened, as if he were pleased to be the first doctor honest enough to break the news to me.

"And yet, you're certain I should get a stent," I said. "So, the risk of a stent must be less than the risk of being on Coumadin."

"Man!" That grin again. I was asking for it. "You want me to play God."

"I assure you I don't."

He wasn't the first doctor who had made such a claim, but he was the first to seem so disappointed when I denied it.

He squirmed in his tweed sport coat.

"I'm forty-four," he said. "We're the same age, man." I wasn't sure where he was going with this, though I figured he was aligning us in time, tossing out a "man" here and there to change the setting, to get us out of the office and into a bar, or a mess hall. He took a deep breath. "Look. The reason for not putting in the stent has been technical, right? You told me that at Penn they were cautious because they were afraid a stent was unsafe."

I nodded. True enough.

"I want you to see my top IR guy, Dr. McMann. If he looks at the scans and decides that, for him, the procedure is low-risk, then

I want you to get a stent."

I didn't challenge him with the question that came to mind. *If I'm literally sailing into uncharted waters, would I feel more confident with the captain who shows caution or with the one who brags of the ease with which he'll sail his ship?* I didn't confess the sense of disloyalty I brought with me or that this feeling had transformed into fierce loyalty toward my team back at Penn.

It was too late, anyway. Anders had put the fear of God into me. I'd scheduled the appointment to see Dr. McMann—a stupid prospect, I realized, since Dr. Trerotola represented, for me, the last word on any medical decision I might make.

As I drove back towards center city, Bruce's album turned dark and slow, with the song "My Depression" and, as I neared home, the ghostly "We Are Alive."

I sat in my car outside my house and called Dad with a full report. Mom, in the background, said that if she were in my shoes, she wouldn't let Anders's hands on her. My dad laughed. "Let's just forget the whole thing happened. Cancel the appointment with McMann. We're not going back there. We'll see Pochettino in June and take it from there."

"He might be going to Mayo soon," I said.

"*Who* might be going to Mayo?"

"Pochettino."

"You're kidding."

"Anders let it slip."

There was a pause. Dad and I were thinking the same thing.

He said, "Well, then, we'll have our excuse to take a trip to Minnesota."

• • •

The first PET-scan since chemo was clear. Dr. Schuster said, "Don't break out the champagne for five years—you can feel confident after two."

"Confident after *two?*" Vana wiped her tears and chuckled. "Oh, thanks a lot."

We told him about my visit with Dr. Anders, who'd urged putting in a stent and getting off Coumadin.

Dr. Schuster said, "You don't get a stent to avoid Coumadin. My father's been on Coumadin for thirty years. Anyway, maybe Pochettino will lower the dosage in June. Who knows, you might be able to come off it altogether. At the very least, another drug will be coming out sooner or later, something less dangerous."

"So it *is* dangerous," Vana said. "See? What about angioplasty?"

"It seems like a promising option," he said. "You need to ask Trerotola."

"What about flying?" she asked.

"Flying?"

"We want to go to Florida," she said, "but we're concerned about cabin pressure or atmospheric pressure or whatever kind of pressure, you know, because of the narrow SVC and the anti-coagulated blood."

He smiled. "Go on vacation. See you in June."

• • •

We flew to Naples. We stayed in a house on the bay, blocks from the beach. The house was owned by a friend of Vana's boss who'd heard about the year we'd had. He'd called and told us to cancel our reservation at the hotel, and to use his car instead of renting one. Our first night there we slept ten hours and woke to sunshine gleaming on the surface of the swimming pool outside the bedroom windows. We spent the morning on the deck, the afternoon on the beach. We cruised in an '86 Mercedes convertible, down wide streets canopied by giant palm trees. It was not difficult to pretend that this was the beginning of life back to normal—as if this paradise were normal.

In a restaurant, Vana and I spied an old couple hunched over an art portfolio, which the man had dug out from the shoulder bag draped on his chair. The woman gently admired one image after another, letting out quiet gasps that evidently pleased the man. Their mouths and fingers moved in subtle ways that only the two of them could translate. Vana and I exchanged embarrassed, hopeful glances.

• • •

In April, I was glad to be back to work, to witness students in action, to be in action myself, to see their eyes light up, their creative minds ignited, as mine was.

Teachers met me with warm smiles. They knew the story. Not much needed to be said. The kids didn't ask questions. They knew I had cancer; that was about it. A girl I'd never taught before called out to me in the hallway, "Hey, Mr. Zervanos, I heard you, like, died." I grinned and showed her my palms, proof of a false rumor. I was back, but not from the dead, exactly.

I had to choke back tears at a pep rally, standing at the edge of the gym floor, sunshine beaming through large windows, a thousand kids shrieking with joy. At times like this I was dumbfounded by the miracle of life, and I did not want to lose this feeling. *I am so happy to be here right now,* I thought, so keenly aware of the alternative. I thought of the Bruce Willis character in *The Sixth Sense,* identifying with the agony of one day realizing that you're a ghost of your former self and that you haven't really been present for the life you think you've been living. In my version the twist was that I woke up to the overwhelming realization that I was *not* dead, but alive, understanding what a fine line existed between here and the other side.

• • •

Months later, in September, on the first day of school, Mal, still fighting pancreatic cancer, sat holding his cane and told me that one of the reasons *he* came back was that he'd heard *I* was back, and he figured that if I could do it, he could do it, too. I told him that I, *too,* had thought of *him* when I was going through it all last year and that a good report about him had always encouraged me. Each morning he sat at a table in the rotunda calling out his welcome, "Good morning!" as well as his warning—as students and I, huffing it from the parking lot, rushed in just before the bell. "Watch your time!"

In February, on the day after he announced his excellent PET-scan results, bellowing about what a beautiful day it was, Mal died at home at his desk with a cigar burning and The Grateful Dead playing on his stereo. The principal's sorrowful voice interrupted first period, just as we turned our attention to Walt Whitman. *All goes onward and outward, nothing collapses . . . And to die is different from what any one supposed, and luckier . . .*

The principal asked me to give the eulogy at the memorial service held in the school's auditorium. I stood silent at the podium for two full minutes, just trying not to lose it, imagining our roles reversed, Mal at the podium and me gone. During my choked-up delay, I felt strangely at ease in the company of my colleagues and Mal's students, who waited patiently. I marveled at, and finally broke, the silence, which seemed to have brought us peace, more than any words ever would.

• • •

In May, I hiked up the museum steps and around to the back, to the plateau that overlooked the river. I decided to pick up speed, to move faster than the usual walking, and before long I broke into a slow jog, pushing my limits. It felt too good to stop, despite feeling rattled. For the first time since last summer, I was running, in the unworn sneakers I'd bought days before going to the hospital.

I rejoined the gym across the street. When the twenty-something manager casually asked about the reason for my hiatus, I smiled. "Health reasons."

"Oh, what kind of health reasons? Were they fitness-related?"

I should have anticipated that she might inquire further, given the general purpose of a gym, and the role of professional trainers.

"I had cancer—and surgery, which saved my life but also left me with limited circulation."

She smiled sheepishly. "I can waive the initiation fee."

I tested my endurance on the stationary bike, at first for thirty minutes, then for an hour. It felt invigorating to sweat so profusely for the first time since waking up drenched from post-surgical fevers, not to mention the whole summer of night sweats before the diagnosis. Encouraged, I headed for the light dumbbells and did curls. I went to the water fountain and bent over for a sip. I stood back up, and *whoah,* I steadied myself on a nearby machine and twisted to find the wall. I was cold and starry-eyed. I anticipated waking up seconds later on the floor. *I should stop,* I thought. *Go home.* But when the feeling passed, I headed to the fly-press machine. I inserted the pin under a thin stack of weights; on second thought, I pulled the pin, leaving just the ten-pound weight. One push and the blood backed up. I cashed in my chips and split. I told myself I never liked lifting weights anyway.

That's what I told myself about running, too. After three days of jogging along the Parkway, my heart developed a strange palpitation. My head felt clogged, as if a cork were stuck in the bottleneck. I made an appointment at Penn. They ran a battery of tests. EKG. Echocardiogram. The nurses pushed me on the treadmill—it was the only way to get a true result, they said, as I huffed and puffed. Later, the cardiologist concluded that last week I must have simply overworked the system, but apparently a few days' rest was all I'd needed because now everything seemed normal. Still, he was fascinated by my case history and admittedly baffled. I asked him about the possibility of doing angioplasty, opening things up in there, and getting off Coumadin. He said, "Let's not take risks when you're doing so well. It hasn't been that long since the surgery, so your anatomy is still adjusting. This may take time." He recommended avoiding running, at least for now. I told him I never loved running anyway.

Later, I walked out to the Parkway and climbed the Art Museum steps. Summer was near. At the top, I caught my breath and took in the view.

25

PSYCHO-SOCIAL ACCELERATION

I was bending over to get something in the pantry when I heard Vana in the kitchen asking, "Are you all right?"

The grunts and groans that broadcast my physical discomfort undercut my desire to face this frustration on my own. My exhausted sighs had become as involuntary as the tingling in my jaws and the metallic taste in my mouth when the head flooded to its limits—my signals to give whatever I was doing a rest. I rushed to tie a Hefty bag spilling over with recyclables, such a simple task that had me on the brink of exploding—not with blood from the ears or anything as horrible as that, but with a furiously growled curse followed by a hurled object.

I'd wondered if the creator of the Incredible Hulk had secretly inflicted the superhero with SVC syndrome, which would explain everything—the cold stare, the dread he felt for his imminent transformation, and the warning, *"Don't make me angry. You wouldn't like me when I'm angry."*

This time, when Vana asked me if I was all right, I tossed the Hefty bag to the floor, mission unaccomplished, and yelled, "I'm fine!"

"It doesn't sound like it."

When she opened the door, I felt accused, not to mention dizzy and out of breath, leaning back against the wall, getting my bearings.

She asked, "Then why are you making those sounds?"

I understood that she meant to convey sympathy, or to discourage activity that caused me such discomfort. I understood that we had been here before and we would be here again, and that each time provided me the opportunity to become a better, kinder, more patient person.

And yet I snapped, "Because my head feels like a fucking stuffed tomato!"

She stared at me, a stranger, and said, "Either you call or I call."

She meant Dr. Brotman, my old therapist, whose office I hadn't visited since long before we got married.

This wasn't the first time she'd given me this advice, but now I knew she meant business because she was willing to make the call herself, which meant we were going together.

"I'll call," I said.

• • •

"The best marriages need some adjusting eventually," my friend Robin told me. She said it was impressive that Vana and I had made it this long without needing therapy. "Most couples are divorced by now," she said, "or at least cheating on each other." I joked that we'd gotten put on hold, thanks to cancer.

"This has been a long time coming," Vana told Dr. Brotman at our first appointment. She explained that a lot of what we needed to discuss went back to issues brewing from before I got sick. Pre-cancer stuff.

He quickly corrected her, "There is no pre-cancer anymore. That stuff would have been dealt with in a way different from the way it will be now. There is only post-cancer. For both of you."

I spent the next twenty minutes telling him the short version of what I'd gone through, starting with the day the neck veins swelled up and that first night in the ER and then the time Dr. Woo told me that what little time I had left would be marked by disability, disfigurement, et cetera.

Dr. Brotman teared up. "You two have been through a lot."

I went on to tell him that, on the other hand, I had never experienced such joy before, such a sense of awareness, presence—all that stuff you hear about, I said, though I didn't mean to diminish it. It's a rush, I told him, sometimes literally, a rush, of lightness to the head, an actual tingling in the spine as I'm walking and looking at the trees and the sky overhead. I have to hold back tears at the thought that I'm here, I can't believe I'm here, God, I'm so lucky to be alive. I'll be so moved by a thought or a moment, I told him, that lately I've been narrating into my iPhone, right there on the sidewalk, sometimes with tears pouring out and people passing by, and I'll record these fragments. Just the other day I was walking by the Barnes Museum and I'm looking at this magnificent building and the flowers and the people inside the windows with their faces aimed at paintings by Matisse, Renoir, and Cezanne, and it just hits me that I'm here and that I'm walking by this place and having this experience and I break out my phone, hit record, and say, "We are all walking miracles." Honestly, it's good that I'm not experiencing these moments and these feelings all the time because I'd be overwhelmed with happiness all day long, at the thought or sight of every minor thing, like a stop sign, or, the other day, I just sat there with Nikitas on my lap, on the sidewalk at our front door, and we watched these two men chopping down a tree on our neighbor's property. Nikitas was completely mesmerized; he didn't want to miss a second of it, and I didn't want to miss a second of it either, watching these two men. I'd never seen anything like it. For hours, from the time these guys climbed to the top and were cutting down branches, till dusk, when they were grinding away at the stump, we just sat there, the two of us, Nikitas in my lap, asking questions and pointing, and I was answering him and pointing, too, soaking in the whole experience.

I stopped myself, seeing how I'd been talking for so long. "Sorry."

Vana gave me a blank stare.

Dr. Brotman explained that some of what I'd been experiencing was not uncommon for older people, in their seventies and eighties, say, as their friends are dying and they begin to face their own mortality. "There's a term for this," he said, "when it occurs in a younger person like you. It's called *psycho-social acceleration*. It can come as a result of an accident or illness, and it accelerates the development of perspective of the younger person."

"See?" Vana let out. "This is the problem! *He's* experiencing a rebirth, and *I'm* going crazy!"

Dr. Brotman grinned. When he saw Vana return his smile, he chuckled. "You're right. His positive attitude can't be making this any easier on you."

Vana elaborated. "I think catastrophic thoughts all day long." She looked at me. "I think of you having a heart attack on the bike at the gym or wrecking on 95 on the way to work or Nikitas drowning at day care or getting hit by a car or my mother dying alone in her house—"

"You think of other people's deaths, not your own," I interrupted, thinking I might be on to something profound.

"*Believe* me," Vana said drolly.

She recalled how we almost hadn't gone to Florida because she'd feared the plane would go down. She said she'd flown, finally, because she needed sunshine, needed to get the hell out. She said she *still* needed to get out. She felt trapped, shut in, by her fears.

Dr. Brotman said he'd been reading Nate Silver's latest book about evaluating risk versus uncertainty, probability versus possibility.

Vana nodded. She got his point.

He said, "We've got some work to do."

• • •

That night Nikitas's bedtime routine regressed further. Vana provided a bowl of cookies, sang more songs. The crib was filled with stuffed animals, beyond the three-animal limit. When he cried, she returned to his room, rocked him to sleep like an infant. "Don't leave me," he said to his mother, as he'd been saying nightly, as if he were trying to break her heart. Vana couldn't bear to hear his plea, any more than I could. When she left, he was at it again, and eventually it was my turn to go in there. "I will never leave you," I told him.

The next morning, I came downstairs to cheers of "Daddy!" When I went to hug Vana, she was silent. When I asked what was the matter, she confessed she was mad at her parents for not having comforted her or talked with her about her fears when she'd first faced them, specifically in 1986, when they took her to see *Mask*, the movie starring Cher as the mother of a severely deformed boy who dies from his rare condition.

"Why did they take me to that? And then why didn't we talk about it?"

"It's not too late," I suggested. "You should tell them. Or we could watch it again, together." I was kidding, she realized, and laughed. "I'm serious," I said, and now maybe I wasn't kidding. I wanted to do what I could to alleviate her fears.

The next week at therapy we got into details. Vana talked about what she saw as my delay tactics, my neglecting responsibilities, or at least being slow to the punch, to check for fevers or to prepare dinners, for example. This line of concern was about fairness and balance, Dr. Brotman reasonably observed. And about Vana's exhaustion, given our new roles—particularly my diminished one—after she'd been an executive for the last eight months. This wasn't just about balancing our roles in the household, either. This was about balancing sympathy with anger, which was compounded by lack of sleep, at least when the kid was up with a fever in the middle of the night.

I thought, *I've got this figured out. This week, cook dinner, give Nikitas Tylenol if he wakes up with a fever. Good session.*

Outside on the sidewalk, Vana didn't return my hug. She said, "This is difficult for me."

In our third session Dr. Brotman reminded us that we'd been talking about fairness and balance last week. Vana dived in with a recent example of an experience that had frustrated her this week when she'd had to instruct me to cook ravioli and edamame beans. She didn't want the control, she explained. I explained that I would have prepared dinner with or without the detailed instructions, that she was asserting control unnecessarily. "Not that I mind the instructions," I said. "I was going to cook ravioli anyway, and edamame beans, or maybe it would have been peas, or carrots."

Vana erupted, "This is bullshit!" and I thought she was about to storm out. "These details are irrelevant!"

Dr. Brotman said to her, "Okay, we're off-track. Get us on-track."

I was in awe of his ability to gently redirect the flow.

Vana collected herself, thought before she spoke.

"This is *not* what this is about," she plainly stated.

Dr. Brotman and I waited for her to tell us what this *was* about. The room remained silent for at least a full minute.

Vana started sobbing. I knew the sound of this cry; it was a rare sound that rose from the depths where she stored her truest pains. I was tempted to console her, but I didn't want to interfere with, or influence, whatever was developing inside herself right now.

"This is about me feeling alone," she said. "It's about me *fearing being* alone . . ."

My heart sank.

. . . *if you die,* she meant.

"Sorry," she whispered.

I couldn't give her guarantees, and I knew that was not what she wanted to hear anyway.

Still, I whispered, "I'm better now." I didn't sound convinced—or convincing.

We, all three of us, wanted to believe this was true. I wouldn't have minded hearing a guarantee myself. *Of course you're better now—all that is over.* Nobody said anything.

"I'm here," I said.

"This is about my feeling insecure," she said. "When I have to be the one to cook dinner or I have to be the one to get the thermometer to take Nikitas's temperature at three in the morning, it makes me feel alone, it makes me fear being alone. Like, this is how it would be." She paused. "This is how it's been, for a long time. That's why I need you to do these things."

I dimly observed, "So all that stuff about edamame beans versus peas, or—"

"Yes! I just need you to do it. I just need you—" She stopped herself. She didn't want to have to explain anymore, to instruct—that was the whole point here. I got it, or so I thought.

"It's okay," Dr. Brotman said. "We don't need to figure all of this out today. We're just scratching the surface, of a lot of things."

And I was thinking, *Wait, didn't we just figure it out?* I was ready to get to work. Cook dinner, give the kid his medicine . . .

Vana nodded, mirroring Dr. Brotman's encouraging smile.

For the first time I felt outside all of this, feeling afraid myself, afraid for what I was failing to understand.

He said to her, "What do you think you need to do?"

"Express myself. Let my guard down. This stuff goes way back. It's about trust."

He nodded. "This is about true intimacy."

She nodded.

They looked at me.

I chimed in, "I'll try to make you feel secure, rather than just passively accept your instructions, even when I'm happy to get them."

She gently smiled. "I don't want to get you down. You're so positive."

"You're not getting me down."

That night before bed I announced that I felt the pain in my ankle returning. She looked at me, puzzled, because I was smiling as if at good news.

"Remember, last year," I said, "when I slipped and sprained my ankle? Well, the whole time I was sick I never felt the pain. I forgot about it completely, or it was actually gone. Now the cancer's gone, and the ankle pain is back."

She was sitting on the bed, an amused grin growing on her face. She teased, "Your back fat is back, too."

I twisted to see it in the mirror. I clenched a fistful and laughed. "Hey, look at that."

She shook her head.

Later, in bed, she cried: "Am I guarded?"

"No," I said. "I don't feel that way."

She wanted to believe me, but my reassurance was beside the point.

"I'm sorry," she said.

"I'm sorry, too."

We were lying there, embracing, but there were lifetimes between us.

26

THANK YOU FOR SAVING MY LIFE, BY THE WAY

For two hours we had been in the waiting room and were now in the exam room—my parents, Vana, and I. The nurse practitioner arrived, one we'd never met; nice guy, asked a few questions about how I'd been, said a few things we already knew—you'll have to stay on Coumadin, your SVC probably isn't going to open up any farther. He said Dr. Pochettino would be in soon, and he exited. Dad said he never let a patient wait more than a half hour. Vana said she was going to have to get going soon to pick up Nikitas from day care, which closed at six. I reminded them that today was Dr. Pochettino's last day at Penn and that he'd never made us feel rushed in all the visits he'd had with us. Today, he must be taking his time with each patient, saying goodbye.

He arrived after 5 p.m., his eyes and smile as soothing as ever. He said my CAT-scan from last week looked the same and we should not expect the SVC's narrowing to change, for better or worse. Collaterals were forming, he said, that was clear enough. For example, the azygous vein appeared enlarged, so it was picking up some slack. As he went on in some detail, the list of questions in my head vanished, as he provided the essential information.

He reminded us that there was a one-percent chance of having a "bleeding event" on Coumadin—anything from having a nosebleed to having something heavy land on me. He grinned. But no stent was necessary, despite the advice of Dr. Anders.

I said, "He scared the hell out of me."

Dr. Pochettino smiled warmly. "He was always a black-and-white guy, and this is not a black-and-white situation. He served in Afghanistan, a military guy."

I understood: he'd been influenced by combat; his strength lay in being decisive under pressure, in using the available weapons, while we had taken a calculating, nuanced approach.

Vana looked at her watch and announced she had to leave. In a rush, she said, "Thank you," and smiled sheepishly, sensing the inadequacy of this frazzled farewell. But maybe it was for the best, a sentiment conveyed through her downcast, teary eyes. She might not be able to handle the full goodbye without losing it.

"Don't forget to ask about angioplasty," she said to me and my parents. "Sorry I have to go."

"No problem," said Dr. Pochettino.

She shook his hand and headed out.

Dad promptly asked about alternatives to a stent. Dr. Pochettino agreed that angioplasty could be a useful option. He encouraged me to make an appointment with Dr. Trerotola, but not until at least September, after we established a new baseline, a new normal.

That smile again. We knew what he was about to say. I was already nodding, as if to give him my blessing, or to forgive him.

"You know I'm leaving for the Mayo Clinic."

We would be in touch, he said, through email or whatever. Penn had hired a new cardiovascular surgeon to fill his position. He wrote down the name of the young man who, technically, would be his replacement. I understood that Dr. Pochettino was following protocol. He looked at me. "There is no one to take my place." I nodded. He was being modest. But he was also warning me. No one here could have done what he did for me. He added, "We're all still learning from you on this."

I gave him an envelope with a card inside, along with a small, wrapped box containing a green metal LOVE sculpture, a token of Philadelphia, one I imagined on a shelf in his new office in Rochester—perhaps right next to the alabaster bust of Hypocrites my mother handed to him. Dr. Pochettino was standing before us with our gifts in his hands. My mom began to cry. She hugged him. My dad choked out, "Thank you for our son." Tears slid down his cheeks as he embraced Dr. Pochettino, whose confident expression still reassured me. When we hugged, he said to me quietly, "I think you're going to be all right."

Together we all exited the room into the quiet, empty hallway. The nurses' station was vacant, as was the large waiting room. There was no one else in sight. I was his last patient. It was past six o'clock on Friday. Tomorrow he was leaving for Minnesota. His wife had already moved, he'd told us; his sons would be joining them after they finished the school year. Before we turned the corner, I looked back to see him, in his dark blue suit, our gifts in his arms, disappearing behind swinging double doors.

"Thank you for saving my life, by the way," I said.

My parents chuckled.

My mom asked, "How do you feel?"

"Good," I said.

My dad said, "I would have liked to read that card you gave him."

"I knew you would." I handed him the folded photocopy I pulled from my pocket.

My mom said, "I hope the bust wasn't too big."

"It was perfect," I said.

My dad pocketed the piece of paper and rested his hand on my shoulder. My mom clutched my arm. As we exited the hospital, I was thinking of the quote on the cover of the card I'd given him, from Louis L'Amour, whose cowboy novels I used to devour as a kid.

"There will come a time when you believe everything is finished; that will be the beginning." I imagined him back in his office, at his desk, opening the card.

Dear Dr. Pochettino,

You told me, "There is always hope," and in an instant there was hope, no matter what would happen. Just hours before, we had hit the bottom, and we were preparing for the end of life, and then you gave me, us, new life, a new vision, well before the surgery that extended my physical life. I thank you for your gift, the gift of your great expertise, which is the result of countless personal sacrifices, countless hours of learning, countless generous acts that preceded the one you provided for me. As the son of another great doctor, I know this is true, that I benefitted not from one single act of surgery but from a lifetime of preparation that you experienced up to that day. I was ready for it, with the full confidence that more capable hands did not exist on the planet. Since waking up, I have lived every day with a heightened sense of gratitude and joy, even in the ICU, even in the grips of chemo—I am ecstatic to be alive. I will remember the moment you walked into that hospital room, before you uttered a word—I felt hope: you exuded it, and I was ready to follow you. I wish you continued success and happiness in your journey, and I thank you for the profoundly, miraculously positive influence you have had on me and my family.

Peace and Love,
Jim Zervanos
6-14-12

Back home, Dad said he had meant to take a photograph of Dr. Pochettino and me together but had somehow forgotten, so caught up in the emotion of the scene despite usually being relentless with the camera. There was something beautiful about that, I thought, my father so swept up in the moment that he hadn't thought to document it. But then I was filled with regret myself, wishing he had been as scrupulous as usual—or that *I* had been. For the next twenty-four hours that sense of loss ridiculously expanded and hardened inside me. *How do I not have a single photograph of this man who saved my life?* In my mind I could see him quite clearly as he entered my hospital room for the first time, in scrubs and lab coat, and then as he exited through those swinging doors, in dark suit and purple tie. I told myself that these images would have to suffice as mementos—along with the graft inside my chest. I told myself that I didn't need a stupid picture, and that if there was one thing I had learned from all of this, it was the temporary nature of everything. I had the scar if I needed something *real* to look at, and, if I lived long enough, even that would fade.

· · ·

In a few months Vana was pregnant, and three months later she wasn't. For more than a day she carried something no longer alive inside her. After the procedure, she reported what the doctor had said in a matter-of-fact way. "It's done. It was just broken parts." Neither of us cried. We confessed that maybe our hearts hadn't been in it—as if we'd played a part in the end. We had become, together, too practiced at protecting ourselves from heartbreak.

Within the year, she was pregnant again. We agreed that if it was a girl we would name her Victoria, after her mother. If it was a boy, Alberto, after my surgeon.

A few months later, when we found out it was a boy, I came home and hugged Vana in the kitchen. "Baby Alberto," I said.

She smiled slightly before turning somber. She sort of cried and laughed at the same time, confessing that she was mortified at the thought of being surrounded by boys, and that she hadn't realized how much she'd actually wanted a girl until today. She said she wasn't so sure about the name Alberto anymore. It would make her think of sad things. I reminded her of the happy things, of hope, of life after death. She was silent. I understood that there was more to her reasoning.

She said, "I think about if you're not here, and then the name will represent pure agony."

I nodded. "Okay."

Months passed until we decided on a name for sure; by then it seemed inevitable—

Victor. As in Victoria—Vana's mom. And Victory. Victor Alberto Zervanos. For a month he had bright blue eyes, like those of his namesake and his grandfather on his father's side, before they turned brown.

27

HE'S ALL I'VE GOT, SHE SAID

In mid-July, Sue and Niko hosted Nikitas's birthday party at their house in Lancaster. The sun was shining. Family and friends filled the patio surrounding the pool. Nikitas was ecstatic in his new single-seater plastic car. Vana put a daisy behind his ear. He leaned on the horn, itching to get motoring.

After cake and ice cream, in candy-cane-striped swimming trunks, Nikitas found his way into the pool, with Uncle Niko, who propped him up on an inflated raft. To Sue, I sarcastically remarked, "This should go well." She knew Niko couldn't help pulling a prank on a trusting toddler. She snickered, and, just like that, Nikitas slipped off the raft. In a flash, he was underwater and back out again. Niko had him at the armpits and into his arms. Nikitas didn't let out a peep, let alone shed a tear, apparently too stunned to know any better.

From the far side of the pool, Vana screamed, "God damn it! God damn it!" marching toward the water's edge. "No! No!" she cried, though Nikitas remained safe in Niko's arms. When Sue and I tried to soothe her, she hid behind the veil of her hand, already regretting her reaction. Instead of whisking Nikitas away, she vanished into the bathhouse.

When I approached to hug her—my ally against all threats to our son—she retreated. "I just embarrassed myself in front of everyone!"

"No you didn't," I said. "Everyone understands."

"I'm sick of this! I don't want to be this way!"

"Wait. What way? I—" I was trying to follow her train of thought.

"Where *were* you? Why is it always *me!*"

I wanted to comfort her. I wanted to defend myself. "I'm on your side," I said, but it made no difference. "I was right there—"

She snapped, "Don't you understand? When I see something like that happen, I think, He's all I've got!"

The words landed like a blow to the chest. I was speechless, literally on my heels. *We're beyond this,* I thought. And then I thought, *We are not beyond this.*

"I'm alive," I said. "You've got me."

The words were hollow. I was back against the counter. I felt like a ghost, as if I were already gone, or as if I hadn't yet returned from where I'd been.

She drifted away.

I found her out by the pool.

She said, "I'm sorry for blaming you for how I feel."

"It's okay," I said. "I'm here for you. I'm going to be here."

She nodded gratefully. I waited for her to say more. *You are here. Yes. I've got you.* But she was silent. I told myself, *Don't expect too much from her. She's been through enough.*

In my mind I kept hearing, *He's all I've got!*

Heading back to Philadelphia that night, with Nikitas sleeping in the back seat, I asked if she remembered what she'd said to me.

She was driving. She kept her eyes aimed on the dark highway.

I said, "Let's just try to be kind to each other."

She was silent.

"Do you want that?"

More silence.

"I was just being rhetorical." I waited. "So, you *don't* want to be kind to each other?" I was asking for it. "What is going on here?" I was prodding at something vague and dangerous. "Hello?" After a long moment, I asked, "Do you love me?"

Finally she spoke. "Just stop."

"You can't say it?"

"Will you please stop?" She glared at me in the darkness.

I leaned against the door. "I can't believe this." I imagined flicking the handle, spilling out onto the highway, rolling into the weeds, and lying there. Dying there.

At home, we stood at opposite ends of the living room. I was waiting to hear something from her to repair this broken night.

"I love you," she said, the words sad and tired.

And then we were back at the pool again.

I reminded her, "'He's all I've got,' you said." I imagined the two of them on their own. "You don't think you've got me?"

She said, "I'm not sure of anything."

"You want a divorce?"

She sighed. "I've thought about it."

She seemed already gone, away from our headaches and sorrows. I lowered myself to the floor, depleted, curling inward, and somehow also outward, toward a dark and empty future without her. I tried to comprehend what this would mean now.

Minutes passed. She crawled to the floor and wrapped her arm around me. "I won't leave you," she said. We lay there, wounded. She let out no sound, while the sorrow poured out of me. Our pain was about much more than either of us could know.

• • •

The next morning the house was quiet. No one uttered a word until after noon. Vana said she needed to return to normalcy but didn't know how to get back there. We talked options. She liked the idea of getting away. I suggested Cape Cod, Cape May, a spa, anywhere away from me and Nikitas to do whatever she needed to do. She said her mom had told her to come to Lancaster. But no, she said, that wasn't quite what she wanted. What she really needed was *not* to go anywhere, and definitely not to stroll on a beach or dine alone in a fancy restaurant. What she needed, she said, was to be here, while Nikitas and I went away for a few days, maybe a week. She needed to dig in the garden, cook in her own kitchen, occupy this space that was her own home, as if it were two years ago, before any of this happened.

At therapy we talked about the birthday party and the aftermath. Dr. Brotman suggested that Vana express the anxiety before it manifested as anger. "You've been very successful in your life at *controlling* your anxiety," he told her, "which is fine *out there in the world*—as a way of functioning—but not with your husband, not with your inner circle. Here, you have to let Jim in, let him comfort you, provide reassurance."

I nodded vigorously. I tried to read Vana's silence. Then I asked, "Why does the anxiety manifest as anger—directed at me?"

Dr. Brotman answered, "It's complicated. She prepared herself for your not being here. 'He's all I've got,' she said, remember? Now you're here." *For now.* He let the point sink in, before he continued. "So it's protect, control." He said to Vana, "He's not going to reject you for expressing your vulnerability—the opposite. He's going to embrace you, comfort you."

She nodded but seemed unconvinced.

"Absolutely," I said. And then, "Wait. That's what this is about? Fear of rejection? *I'll* reject *you* before *you* reject *me?*"

He grinned. "You have a lot of good questions. A lot to think about."

In the car heading home, Vana suggested that I go to Lancaster alone for the weekend and that Nikitas stay with her in Philly.

"*Me* alone?" I was baffled by this reversal.

Driving, she kept her eyes aimed straight ahead.

I was trying to follow.

I said, "Now you don't even want to be *alone?*"

"I just want to relax in my own home."

I looked out the passenger window, down Walnut Street, toward Rittenhouse Square buzzing with life. "You just spent the last hour talking about how you were an only child, you need your space, you can't remember the last time you woke up and just enjoyed a solitary cup of coffee."

"How am I supposed to relax being here alone all weekend? What's the point?"

I waited for eye contact that didn't come. "The point is to face your fears. To let go. So we can try to move forward."

"I don't want to face my fears!" Her hands wrung at the steering wheel. "That's not why I wanted to do this!"

"So now you're sending me off alone? How is that progress?"

"Forget it! The whole idea is stupid."

We crossed the Parkway, rounding the fountain.

I tried again. "Okay, let's—"

"I don't feel comfortable with any of this. How are you going to take care of him?"

"How am I—? Is that what you're worried about?"

"What about a bath? You can't even give him a bath. You can't bend over to—"

"I won't give him a bath."

"What if he throws up in the car?"

"I'll pull over and clean it up."

She huffed.

I said, "I want to be with him. I've been looking forward to this. I won't let him out of my sight. I promise."

We were a block from home.

"I'm just not sure it's worth the anxiety, being alone here, thinking about you two there. What am I going to do?"

We passed the Whole Foods, the Starbucks.

"That's one of the benefits of this whole being-home-alone thing—you might just miss us. *Me.*" I tried a smile.

She parked outside our door. The car was quiet. She turned to me. "I need you to reassure me he'll be okay."

"He'll be fine. We're going to have fun together."

"I think about *you, too.*"

I mirrored her smile. "I'll be fine."

She let out a deep breath. "Okay."

"This will be good for you—us."

She nodded. "But not Friday. You can leave Saturday, after lunch. And then be back before it gets dark on Sunday."

So, this was the plan. Apart for twenty-four hours. It was a start.

28

ANGIOPLASTY

In August I had my appointment with Dr. Trerotola to discuss angioplasty. By now I was convinced that this ballooning procedure would be my way back to living normally. Now that the graft had healed, we would just go in there and open that SVC right back up.

When Dr. Trerotola arrived in the exam room, lean and smiling, in his white lab coat, he seemed delighted to see me and a bit puzzled. "I'm surprised to see you're not puffed up!"

"Why?"

"When I saw your name on my patient appointment list, I assumed you were having symptoms. In fact, I emailed a cardiovascular surgeon to ask if it would be okay to do angioplasty on a graft."

For a moment, I was relieved it wasn't the emergency he'd anticipated.

He said, "I've never done a stent or angioplasty on an SVC graft."

In the pregnant pause that followed, I realized that the relief I'd been hoping for was not in the cards, at least not anytime soon. I was embarrassed, not just disappointed, for the assumptions I'd made.

He smiled. "So, tell me why you're here."

As diplomatically as I could, I explained that Dr. Pochettino had encouraged me to do angioplasty. I explained how he'd said that, if he were in my situation, he would do it, since it was a very common procedure and low-risk, with high-benefit potential.

Dr. Trerotola nodded. I could see he was measuring his words.

I said, "It wasn't just Dr. Pochettino. It was my dad and other doctors, too."

He sighed. "As an expert in my field, and even just as a doctor, I try not to speak authoritatively on medical matters outside my expertise."

I got the message: these other doctors didn't know what they were talking about.

Dr. Trerotola gave me a firm look. "There is no such thing as a benign angioplasty. I can count on one hand how many venous angioplasty patients never returned for further treatment. The rest were back within six to eight months for more angioplasty and eventually a stent, which leads to clots, which then lead to big problems."

Dr. Woo's angel-of-death speech rang in my ears: one intervention led to another, and then another, and then . . . that's it.

Dr. Trerotola must have seen the dread on my face. "I'm not convinced the SVC is done shaping itself." He was reading the most recent CAT-scan report. "It looks like, at its narrowest, it's still about three millimeters"—about one-fifth the normal measurement.

"Maybe after the graft has healed completely," I said, "after the vein's actual cells have taken over, and the graft has, you know, *resorbed* into the body," as I recalled the process, "would you, then, possibly, reconsider doing the angioplasty?"

He grimaced. "The graft will always be a foreign substance. Collagen. Dead tissue," he explained—contrary to my longtime understanding. He clarified. The so-called resorption of the graft refers to the graft material being replaced by body cells on the *inside* of the graft, which itself moves *outward*. Much healing and manipulation take place, for better and for worse, thus the dramatic narrowing. The bottom line is, the graft is still a graft and always will be. Or put another way, it's not really a vein and never will be.

"You look great," he reassured me. "Normal."

"I still have symptoms. When I bend over, and whenever I—"

"Show me," he said.

I bent over, pretending to towel-dry my feet. When I stood upright, my face wasn't as flush as I wanted it to be.

He said, "No one should be bending over like that, anyway."

"I know. I just—"

"It's bad for your back."

"I can't lift weights, not even the single plate on the machines, and I can't run—"

"You don't need to lift weights."

He asked me to lift my shirt to see evidence of collateral veins. I lifted my shirt to my armpits. He was surprised not to see blue veins. There must be collaterals, was the theory, but ordinarily they'd be protruding right there on the chest wall. "They might still form," he said, and then, still perplexed, he said, "Let's take a look at the CAT-scans."

He reeled them up, right there on the computer at the corner desk.

I asked, "Why do you think there aren't collaterals visible on my chest?"

He shrugged. "Who knows?"

Together we looked at the three-dimensional images. He was amazed, as I was—just as we'd been almost a year ago, on the day of the venogram—at how narrow the SVC appeared up close, like some kind of wormhole astronomers can't explain.

"At worst," he said, "there's no change. At best, maybe it's slightly more open, just over three millimeters."

He zoomed in, as in a video game.

The vein narrowed to a dot smaller than a Tic Tac. I squinted, shaking my head, incredulous. "It's hard to imagine any blood making it through there at all."

"I can't say I understand it either. But—" He made sure I was looking at him, not at the screen. "We don't have to understand it. It's working." He shut off the computer. We stood eye-to-eye. "Let's not try to fix what's not broken."

He had me feeling as though I were part of the decision-making process. I was grateful to be included. "Absolutely," I said.

I wanted him to know that I was doing well, despite the limitations I'd described. I wanted him to know, too, that I was grateful for what he'd once again had the good sense *not* to do. I announced, "I've managed to get my heart rate down from 98 to 78, just from riding the bike at the gym. Sixteen miles in sixty minutes, almost daily. No one knew why my heart rate was so high—whether it was the chemo or the narrow SVC—but the advice was exercise."

"See? There you go." He grinned. "You don't need to run, either."

I tried to smile. "I let my hopes get too high. I had visions this procedure would restore me to normal. I don't know if what you're telling me is good news or bad news."

"This is all good news," he said. "The body forms what it must, because it must, and your body is evidently functioning well as it is. Let's give this another six months and see where we are. When you see Schuster and get your next PET, let's get a scan of the graft." He gave me his card. "Hopefully you'll never have to call me, but if you do, it's no hurry. There will be time, and I will do whatever I have to do the next day, or *that* day."

"I appreciate your caution," I said.

"I'm not cautious." He waited for my full attention. "I actually have a reputation for being a risk-taker."

He didn't need to explain the difference between *risky* and *reckless.*

We shook hands.

End of story. For now.

• • •

Back home, Vana and I hugged, united in our disappointment. "Please be okay," she said.

"Please be with me no matter what," I said.

"Okay."

The next morning, she woke me and said, "Can you go downstairs? Nikitas is in the bathroom on the toilet, and he doesn't want to get out."

When I got down there, the door was closed. I opened it. He was standing there, with his pants at his ankles, pointing. "I did it! I pooped." And he had. There it sat. He flushed it and pranced heroically in the nude.

Vana came downstairs dressed for work. "How do you feel?" she asked.

"A little depressed," I said. "Something was taken away yesterday. But I understand it was something I never had. I mean, not since, you know—"

We both teared up, prepared to let go of that hope for a magical procedure to make me normal again. We held each other extra long.

"Please be careful," she said.

"Of course," I said.

"No, I mean, I had a dream that you were shot in the face—"

"What? Jesus!" I laughed. "Remember when you asked your mom to keep her morbid dreams to herself?"

"You were okay!" she said. "It was just in the cheek or something."

"Oh, well, that's lucky!"

She laughed and rushed off to work, while I took my time with Nikitas, in no hurry to take him to school. He tuned right in. Or maybe I had tuned in to him. He was one step ahead of me as usual.

"Sit right here." He pointed to the kitchen floor. "No friends, no school," he said, and plopped himself in my lap and cooked his letter magnets in the small pot with the glass lid.

"Okay." I kissed his head and watched.

In a minute I managed to get him upstairs, where we sat and moved the train around our bodies on the floor. I asked if he wanted to go to the store before school. "To buy yogurt," I said. That did the trick. We went to the Whole Foods to buy yogurt and peaches; then

I took him to school. He entered the classroom shyly and made his way to the table of kids, his "friends," eating Rice Krispies. I kissed his face and said have a good day.

Outside I felt more alive than I had in months. Such is the effect of facing your mortality. Anyone can grasp the fact that his life is temporary, but there's no substitute for the bittersweet taste of the immediate experience of it. So, for now, this ecstatic feeling of living was back. I swallowed it and looked up, and there was the sun, and the leaves, and all that there was of the future was the bright sidewalk stretching out before me as I set one foot in front of the other—as if this were the last time I would ever have this feeling.

29

NIGHT SWEATS

Two years after it all started, Vana and I rushed to move out of the city and into the suburbs before Victor was due to be born in February. By mid-January, only weeks after we settled into our "new" hundred-year-old house—and only weeks before Victor's delivery date—a relentless series of snowfalls threatened to strand us at home. I'd already spent countless hours pushing the snow blower, keeping the driveway clear for safe passage, pausing frequently to let the backed-up blood in my head return to my heart. Inside the house we found our way among the boxes, lifting and hauling, emptying and hanging; this new life demanded more from my altered physiology than it could handle—a fact I was loath to admit.

And so I found myself, weeks after move-in day, sitting, weary, on Nikitas's bedroom floor, face-to-face with my sister, who set her eyes on me and said, "You seem angry all the time."

This was just after we'd struggled to move a bookshelf and I'd snapped, "Just leave it where it is."

"You have all the reasons in the world to be happy," she said. "Soon you're going to be the father of two sons. You need to make this house a home where your kids feel love, not frustration. Are you depressed? I know you were anxious about the cancer coming back, but you're healthy now."

I sat there, defenseless.

She said, "It's not pleasant to be around you when you're like this. It's too intense. You need a way to relieve the tension. You need to let go."

I recognized the anxiety I'd been storing up and releasing in minor explosions, which I'd believed were private and discreet, or at least ignored and forgotten by others. The tension was all rising to the surface now and becoming lodged in my throat.

Sue was on a roll. "You have a disability. You're going to have to live with these symptoms for the rest of your life. You need to accept that you can't do all the things you used to be able to do. You need to ask for help—"

"From who?" I interrupted. "My eight-months-pregnant wife?"

Sue looked at me tenderly. "You sound like Dad."

I steadied myself. "Sometimes you just have to do what needs to get done."

She leaned toward me, with grave, imploring eyes. "You *need* something. Medication. Or therapy. What are you going to *do?*"

I took a deep breath. "I'm going to wake up tomorrow and keep trying to be a better person."

She smiled patiently, understanding better than I did that sheer willpower would not be enough. She led me downstairs to the kitchen, where our mother and Vana were unpacking boxes, pretending not to know what business Sue and I had just been discussing.

• • •

For several days in a row, I woke up in a soaked T-shirt. At first, I attributed the sweating to the old house's radiator heat, which my body was unaccustomed to. I made this assumption even though night sweats were the number-one symptom to look out for as a sign that lymphoma had returned. Meanwhile, I was due for my two-year PET-scan in three weeks.

We lowered the heat, and with each night that followed it became more difficult to chalk the night sweats up to the radiators or even to poor insulation, even though my side of the bed sat against a cool, dampish wall. Vana offered to trade sides, though being eight months pregnant, she preferred the side near the bathroom. Still, the night sweats persisted. The next night I was back against the wall. At three in the morning Vana heard me sigh as I changed my shirt. We didn't say a word.

In the morning I emailed Danielle Land and asked if I should move up the date of my PET-scan. She wrote back, *Jan 21 is soon, so you can either wait or, if you want, call and ask if there is an earlier appt. Either is fine with us.*

That night I woke up soaked.

The next day I called radiology. When I told the operator I'd been having night sweats, he expedited the schedule change. In four days, I would find out if I had cancer.

I reminded myself of Dr. Brotman's advice, about probability versus possibility. You can alleviate your anxiety by reminding yourself of the difference. After ten straight days of night sweats— after two years of dry T-shirts—it was hard to believe it was only possible, not probable, that the lymphoma was back.

I remembered a year ago, after the one-year post-chemo PET-scan, Dr. Schuster had brought a plate of baklava to the follow-up appointment—three large syrupy triangles on a Styrofoam plate with plastic spoons from a local restaurant. I beamed, "I hope that's celebratory baklava!" He laughed. We feasted—Vana and I, Danielle and Dan and Dr. Schuster. We took pictures, arms draped across each other's shoulders. That night Vana burst into tears on my chest. "Please don't leave me!" These words she'd then felt free to say out loud in the wake of good results. "I've been so worried about you every day." Now I feared we'd celebrated prematurely.

For the next four days until the PET-scan, I was reminded of the body's own mysterious and separate existence, and of the possibility that the end might be drawing near after all. I kept thinking, *There is no time to waste, to live the way I want to live!* And, *How I've screwed up! I keep screwing up!*—as if, by now, after the experience I'd had, I should be living in a constant state of gratitude and generosity. In these moments of heightened awareness, I wanted nothing more than to exorcise all desire and disappointment from my mind and soul. *Why can't I get it right? How many brushes with death do I need?* I thought of the innumerable times my words or actions had hurt others, and the infinite number of times my thoughts had kept me from being truly present in my life. I told myself I should know better. I confessed all of this to Vana one night in bed. I admitted that, when this line of thinking got the best of me, I wondered if maybe I'd been meant to die. If maybe the life-saving surgery had altered the natural path of things. Maybe I should have gone out on top, when I'd reached that pinnacle of life, as I recalled, when I'd been at peace with death and filled with a sense of love and fulfillment that I now feared I would never again attain, let alone sustain. I reminded myself to breathe, just breathe, understanding how I must continuously seek to synchronize my mind and soul with the peace and joy that offered their hands to me at every moment, and how I must continuously forgive myself for failing to grasp them. This was the challenge of a lifetime, I realized, as Vana and I fell asleep in each other's arms.

Driving home from work, the day before the dreaded PET-scan, I was at the intersection a few blocks from the school, talking on the phone with Vana, when in a flash the idea of letting my foot off the brake and drifting into oncoming traffic came to me. The thought frightened me even as it passed. I understood the urge and even wondered how the unconscious, with a stronger push from within, might have the force to lift a foot off a pedal. I understood what it meant to feel so tired and unwilling to go on. And then there was a clearing, and I hit the gas.

The next day, Dr. Schuster's calendar was so packed that he couldn't see me for the customary appointment immediately after the PET-scan to discuss the results. Instead, Danielle promised to email me the next day.

In the twenty-four hours that followed, Vana and I had virtually resigned ourselves to getting the bad news. What else could explain the continued night sweats? Before I went to work the next morning, I emailed Danielle and asked her to call me with the results as soon as possible. At 7 a.m. she wrote back that she would call me on my cell phone as soon as she saw the report. I managed to get through the day at school, teaching, allowing the routine activities to distract me from my fears. A part of my mind, all on its own, kept rehearsing my reaction to Danielle's call. In my imagination, when my phone rang, I excused myself from the classroom. In the hallway I heard her say, "We need you to come in," and I crumpled against the lockers before lowering myself to the floor. I didn't cry; I was too numb, dried out, facing chemo and maybe radiation and the unknown future that suddenly held the increased possibility that I would not be around for the long haul.

Until today I had never gone to the internet, not once in these two and a half years, to look up anything relating to my illness, heeding the advice of the many reasonable people who warned against doing my own research, certain of the horror that would come with my discoveries. Today, I couldn't resist Googling *night sweats*. First on the list of causes? *Stress*.

I took a deep, hopeful breath.

My teacher friend Dave stopped by my classroom after school to see how I was doing. He knew about the news I was waiting for, and about the symptoms I'd been experiencing. I held my hand out flat like a coin and said heads you have cancer, tails you don't. That's how it feels, 50-50. It could go either way.

At 3 p.m. I emailed Danielle and reminded her that I was hoping to hear from her soon. Six students from the lit-mag staff hovered quietly over stories they were reading at a nearby table. Minutes later she replied. I opened the email impulsively and read. *The preliminary report just came back and there is no evidence of lymphoma! I will let you know when the final report is back.* For a moment I didn't physically react, though my mind was processing this information. Then my eyelids welled up, and I let out something like a stifled sneeze, a gasp, a choked-off sob. I felt my body draining of tension I hadn't even known existed. Top cause of night sweats—*stress.*

I headed out into the hallway and walked toward the school's lobby, toward air and sunlight.

I called Vana and told her the news. Her joyful cry was indistinguishable from a sad whimper. "I know, I know," I said. Somehow, for us, for now, joy and sorrow—or at least our expressions of these feelings—had blurred. We listened to the silence between us and around us. We were relieved and thankful, and numb, floating somewhere beyond the pain that we had been preparing ourselves to endure.

I woke up the next morning in a dry T-shirt.

30

ANNIVERSARY

One year to the day since my neck and head first swelled with blood, I thought the best way to commemorate the anniversary would be to take Nikitas to a baseball game. But the Phillies were on the road, in Milwaukee, so we accepted my parents' invitation and drove to the beach house for a few days.

On our first morning there, I walked for an hour, taking in another in a series of audio books. To get the heart rate up, I tried to jog, just a block or two, despite my better judgment, and of course the symptoms flared up. I told myself to give it a rest. I wanted to be healthy, was all. When I got back to the house, I took the bike out and cruised around town for a while longer.

I couldn't stop thinking about that day a year ago, and about the year that had followed. I remembered, an hour before everything changed, sitting at my favorite fountain with Nikitas on my lap, our faces smiling obliviously in the breeze, and a week later lifting Nikitas into the air at the beach, despite my mysterious condition, as if for the last time. I would do everything for those next few weeks as if for the last time. I'd wished only that I would survive to see him grow up and one day throw a ball. I hadn't dared to wish that I would throw the ball back.

When I returned from my bike ride, I took a shower before lunch. The bathroom door opened and Nikitas asked, "What's Daddy doing?" Vana opened the curtain, and Nikitas looked up at me and my shampooed hair. A smile spilled across his face. "Daddy like Superman!" He knew Superman from a small plastic figure with a cape in his toy box. He pointed to the foamy curl pasted to my forehead. "Superman like Daddy."

"Yes!" I replied—*as if.*

At lunch we told Nikitas to drink his milk so he could get big. Persuaded, he gulped at his cup, set it down, and asked, "I'm big now?" We beamed at him. He took another hopeful swig.

After lunch it was time for his nap. "No bed," he said, but without much fuss he was in the bedroom, with his book of choice picked out.

At page one he was reciting, from his magnificent memory, the opening line, "The night Max wore his wolf suit and made . . ." As Max wielded his fork at his little white dog fleeing, Nikitas was grinning, "mischief of one kind . . . and another . . ." Halfway, he yawned, "Let the wild rumpus start!" We sang the songs we'd made up for the wordless pages. When we finished, we positioned the book in the corner of the crib, open to our favorite page, where Max the king is hoisted upon the Wild Things marching through the forest.

I had managed to get past tearing up at every marvelous moment, at every bit of meaningless beauty, though I remained as aware as I could be of the miraculous reality of this life, of the breath that sustained me, of my ever-pumping heart, fast or slow, of my cooperative body with all its confounding mysteries that scans couldn't explain. As Nikitas slept, my dad read at the kitchen table, my mom paged through a magazine in the living room, Vana headed to the post office, and I sat by the window with my laptop, considering what work there was to accomplish. I wondered if, or when, I would ever write about this experience I'd been through. *Too soon,* I decided. Writing about my life was not how I wanted to spend a single moment of it. For the time being, everything else seemed far too important.

· · ·

Back in Philly a few days later, Nikitas and I headed down the street to watch the Little League game at the park. Deep in the outfield, I threw him pitches that he whacked at with his fat plastic bat. He watched the boys on the dirt diamond in the distance and said he was going to play, too, "when I get big." He asked me if I was going to play "when you get small?" *When I get small.* I contemplated the innocent genius of this question. Of course, through eyes that don't know death, life must at some point begin again. "Yes," I lied, "when I get small," and for a moment we existed in a field where time bends back on itself and we grow younger after we've grown older and we get to be here together forever.

BEGIN AGAIN

Three months had passed since the day Vana had laid bare the truth before me and I was seeing stars. Five years since the cancer.

We were once again sitting in Dr. Brotman's office, where we'd been coming weekly.

"Life keeps asking the same question until you answer it," Dr. Brotman said. "And then it asks you a new question."

So many questions had been asked in these past three months that I couldn't begin to guess which question, or questions, he was referring to; which was the *same question* Life kept asking us and, if we had answered it, then which was the *new question* Life was asking us now. Dr. Brotman gave us a moment to ponder all of this. I looked at Vana, who appeared to have all the answers, while I felt as if I knew nothing at all anymore. At once I understood that this was a turning point for me, feeling at ease in this state of not-knowing, which felt something like knowing.

I remembered Vana the summer we started dating, a family event back in our hometown, her walking across the restaurant parking lot toward me, beaming, long skirt swinging, hair swaying, while I aimed my camera, recording a brief video of this girl I already hoped to marry. I remembered us kissing in her apartment, her saying, "I'm not interested in just fooling around," and me saying, "Neither am I," and, not long after that waking up in her bed and telling her that we were going to be together and her asking, "How do you know?" and me answering, "I just know."

Ten years later, here we were, side by side yet divided by the very experiences that bound us together. We had been broken, repaired somewhat, grown stronger, wiser—but separately, and incompletely. We needed to find our way home again. Recognize each other's afflictions. Combine our strengths. Salve our unique wounds.

"You don't know who I am anymore," Vana said to me. She went on to paint a picture of someone who, at work, felt invigorated, animated, appreciated—a thrilling depiction of a woman whose return, or arrival, I longed for at home, where I had failed to recognize the depth of her unhappiness, despite her attempts to reveal it to me.

"Your first marriage is over," Dr. Brotman announced. "The question now is whether you're capable of a second marriage with each other."

We had covered more ground in here than I could ever remember.

"I still think of you getting sick," Vana said. "Of you not being here. I still fear losing you. When you exercise. When I see your face get full and red and puffy."

"You've got a very different perspective," Dr. Brotman reminded me. "You're still enjoying a second lease on life. And you," he said to Vana, "you've had an awakening."

It was true, for better and for worse. While Vana was thriving professionally, I couldn't wait to get home from work. To be with her and the kids. It had been a long time since I'd been distracted by the nagging need to write, to finish the story, the novel, the screenplay, the memoir. All of that had become less important to me. Almost unimportant, compared to what I valued most. Recently I'd even announced for the first time in my life that I was quitting writing, an experiment that lasted two days, long enough to experience the relief—and a distant fear—of knowing I might actually have it in me to free myself from this ordeal of arranging and rearranging words on a page for purposes that often seemed elusive. Meanwhile, Vana was planning on getting her doctorate.

"I just want to start over," she said. All of us rested in the long silence that followed, until she added, "And can we please not come back here for a while?"

A week later we were on a plane headed for New Orleans, a city neither of us had ever visited. Vana had a conference for work, just for the weekend. The kids were home with the grandmoms. The night before the trip Vana had said she was excited to fly. Not just excited to see New Orleans. But to fly. The actual flying. The physical experience of it. My wife, whose fear of flying had once been paralyzing. She was letting go of the past. I was ready to follow her lead. Just before takeoff she took my hand. I returned her bold smile. We were getting to know each other all over again, which made the connection feel all the more thrilling. And a little frightening.

· · ·

Two weeks later I sat in the waiting room for my five-year post-cancer checkup, the break-out-the-champagne appointment I'd been looking forward to—assuming all went well, and there was no reason not to assume. For the past two years, Dr. Schuster had found PET-scans unnecessary, content with bi-annual blood tests and physical exams. I knew from experience that by late afternoon he would be behind schedule, so I'd brought my laptop to continue with the writing I'd recently returned to.

I peeked up and listened to a hip bald woman dressed in black, with high heels and funky, thick-rimmed glasses, on her phone with a friend or family member, fuming about her blood test, how she'd followed doctor's orders and eaten a big steak last night and yet somehow whatever crucial number had dropped even lower. "So I guess tonight I'm going to eat an even bigger steak," she said.

I liked her attitude. Her edge. She wore her baldness as if it had been her style before the chemo. I waited for eye contact that never came. I wanted to tell her to hang in there, not that she needed my encouragement. Then her name was called and she marched out of the waiting room and down the long hallway.

An hour later, I was called back to my exam room where I waited for Dr. Schuster. I sat in the desk chair as the laptop grew warm on my thighs. It was nearly six when I texted my brother to tell him I'd be late for our six-thirty dinner reservation. I scooted my chair across the floor and set my laptop on the exam bed. I was making my way through the memoir, having decided weeks ago to shift it to past tense, to break out of the present, which had created a sense of immediacy that was too much to demand of the reader, and of myself. And so there I was, changing "breathe" to "breathed," "run" to "ran," "live" to "lived," "fly to "flew." It felt good to be telling this story in retrospect, rather than to be bringing it all back to life in the moment.

From behind the door across the hall I could hear a patient asking about iron deficiency and the curative potential of red meat—the hip, bald woman from the waiting room. Dr. Schuster was taking his time to provide the explanation and reassurance she needed.

Another hour passed. I texted John again. He said no problem. He was in no hurry. The advantages of bachelor life, he joked.

Dr. Schuster finally showed up around seven-thirty. He apologized for the delay. I told him I was happy to get some work done. I said my brother and I had postponed our dinner reservation until nine. "I should have you out of here by then," he said, and asked me about my life and family. After examining me, he said, "I don't need to see you again. Unless you're going to miss me too much. How about we say one year from now? Can you wait that long?"

We hugged, and I thanked him for everything.

He said, "Someday when you've lived a long life and I'm looking down from above, I'll say I cured you."

I said, "I'm not against you saying you cured me right now."

"I don't like to use that word." He wouldn't say it again. *Cured.* "I don't want to jinx anything."

"I'm not sure I want to know, but I'll ask anyway. How many people who have what I had—?"

He finished my sentence, "Relapse after five years? It's hard to give a percentage, but let's just say it's way under one percent."

I smiled. "You once told me that after five years my odds of getting it are the same as the general population's."

"That's right." He grinned. "I've got as good a chance as you at this point." He looked once more at the results of my blood work. "Even your liver numbers are low. That's good. Are you drinking enough?" I laughed. He glanced at his watch. "If it weren't so late, I'd have a drink with you and your brother."

Before nine, John and I were toasting to good health, and he asked me how things were going on the home front. We spoke of progress and taking stock of all there was to be grateful for. We recalled the stressful fall we'd both been through. I mentioned the verdict going the wrong way in his big case. "I have my health, and that's all that matters," he said. "I'm not the one sitting at home in a wheelchair, like my client, facing a lifetime of disability." I nodded. After dinner we shook hands out on the sidewalk before parting, John off to his pad in center city, I to my house in the suburbs.

When I got home, Vana and I poured the champagne and made a toast to fresh starts. She gave me a card with a heart on it. In the note she told me she'd do it all over again—*all over again.* "I would too." The house was still. Vana and I sipped and smiled, standing in the bright kitchen, drawn toward the mystery of each other and of the rest of our lives.

ACKNOWLEDGMENTS

This book is, among other things, an expression of my gratitude toward every person named in it. To all of you, I thank you for your love, for your friendship, for your professional care and expertise, all of which saved my life and inspired me to tell this story. Beyond that, my deepest thanks to Robin Black, John Fried, Mike Fitzgerald, Matt Hartin, Alex Lyras, Dan Peterson, Bob Huber, John Pritchard, Lloyd Brotman, and Scott Trerotola, for your extraordinarily insightful and encouraging readings that helped me write this book.

I'd also like to thank many people not otherwise mentioned in these pages who have helped me tremendously to bring this book to life. Dan Loose, your years of friendship, tutelage, and brilliant editing have been one of the great gifts of my life. Dennis and Dot Baumwoll, thank you for continuing my education long after college, in your home, in your letters and emails; Dennis, I can see you grinning, and I miss you. Kelly Simmons, your singularly generous reading pointed the way. Scott Gould, Greg Fields, Lauren Sheldon, Joe Coccaro, and John Koehler, thank you for guiding me and the book to publication at Koehler Books. Dean Fournaris, thank you for your expert counsel. Thank you to my wonderful and amazing writers' group, Julie Odell, Tony Knighton, Kath Hubbard, and

Nathan Long. Noel Lorson and Dave Berk, thank you for your artistic brilliance. Nan Wisherd, thank you for your crucial and ongoing support. Thank you to so many friends for your generous readings along the way, above all Beth Kephart, Bonnie West, Scott Meltzer, Kevin Maness, Brad Mellinger, Diana England, Christine Weiser; and my Penncrest friends, Ben Danson, Rob Simpson, Felicia Quinzi, Steve Silva, Winnie Host, and Carolyn Heaton. Becky Fawcett, thank you for being a bright shining light.

Mom and Dad, thank you for, well, everything.

Thank you, John and Sue—the best brother and sister a little brother could have. The bond I feel with you is beyond blood.

Vana, thank you, I love you, I'm so happy to be here with you. And our boys, Nikitas and Victor—as if I'm not lucky enough—I have you two, too.

CPSIA information can be obtained
at www.ICGtesting.com
Printed in the USA
LVHW111439211122
733705LV00002B/50

9 781646 638178